T0299731

Activity Groups in Family-Centered Treatment: Psychiatric Occupational Therapy Approaches for Parents and Children

Activity Groups in Family-Centered Treatment: Psychiatric Occupational Therapy Approaches for Parents and Children has been co-published simultaneously as *Occupational Therapy in Mental Health*, Volume 22, Numbers 3/4 2006.

Activity Groups in Family-Centered Treatment: Psychiatric Occupational Therapy Approaches for Parents and Children

Laurette Olson, PhD, OTR/L

Activity Groups in Family-Centered Treatment: Psychiatric Occupational Therapy Approaches for Parents and Children has been co-published simultaneously as *Occupational Therapy in Mental Health*, Volume 22, Numbers 3/4 2006.

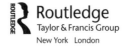

Routledge
Taylor & Francis Group
New York   London

First published by

The Haworth Press, Inc., 10 Alice Street, Binghamton, NY 13904-1580

This edition published 2012 by Routledge
711 Third Avenue, New York, NY 10017
27 Church Road, Hove, East Sussex BN3 2FA

Activity Groups in Family-Centered Treatment: Psychiatric Occupational Therapy Approaches for Parents and Children has been co-published simultaneously as *Occupational Therapy in Mental Health*™, Volume 22, Numbers 3/4 2006.

The development, preparation, and publication of this work has been undertaken with great care. However, the publisher, employees, editors, and agents of The Haworth Press and all imprints of The Haworth Press, Inc., including The Haworth Medical Press® and Pharmaceutical Products Press®, are not responsible for any errors contained herein or for consequences that may ensue from use of materials or information contained in this work. Opinions expressed by the author(s) are not necessarily those of The Haworth Press, Inc. With regard to case studies, identities and circumstances of individuals discussed herein have been changed to protect confidentiality. Any resemblance to actual persons, living or dead, is entirely coincidental.

The Haworth Press is committed to the dissemination of ideas and information according to the highest standards of intellectual freedom and the free exchange of ideas. Statements made and opinions expressed in this publication do not necessarily reflect the views of the Publisher, Directors, management, or staff of The Haworth Press, Inc., or an endorsement by them.

Library of Congress Cataloging-in-Publication Data

Olson, Laurette.
    Activity groups in family-centered treatment : psychiatric occupational   therapy approaches for parents and children / Laurette Olson.
        p. ; cm.
        "Published simultaneously as Occupational therapy in mental health, volume 22, numbers 3/4 2006."
    Includes bibliographical references and index.
    ISBN-13: 978-0-7890-3509-7 (hard cover : alk. paper)
    ISBN-10: 0-7890-3509-X (hard cover : alk. paper)
    ISBN-13: 978-0-7890-3510-3 (soft cover : alk. paper)
    ISBN-10: 0-7890-3510-3 (soft cover : alk. paper)
    1. Family psychotherapy. 2. Occupational therapy. 3. Mentally ill parents. 4. Occupational therapy for children. 5. Parent and child. I. Title. II. Title: Psychiatric occupational therapy approaches for parents and children.
    [DNLM: 1. Occupational Therapy–psychology. 2. Child Psychology. 3. Mental Disorders–therapy. 4. Parent-Child Relations. 5. Parents–psychology. 6. Psychotherapy, Group. W1 OC601N v.22 no.3/4
2006 / WS 350.2 O52a 2006]
    RC488.5.O397 2006
    616.89'156–dc22
                                                                            2006024543

Activity Groups in Family-Centered Treatment: Psychiatric Occupational Therapy Approaches for Parents and Children

CONTENTS

ABOUT THE AUTHOR

Laurette Olson, PhD, OTR/L, is currently Associate Professor in the Graduate Program in Occupational Therapy at Mercy College in Dobbs Ferry, NY, where she teaches courses about small group process, and pediatric and adolescent occupational therapy practice. She also serves as a consultant for occupational therapy program development and supervision at the Alcott Montesorri School and at the Mamaroneck Union Free School District in Westchester County, NY. Over the past 25 years, she has worked with parents and children in both hospital and school-based settings. Over a ten year span, Dr. Olson worked at New York Hospital-Cornell Medical Center, Westchester Division as a staff occupational therapist, supervisor, and program coordinator. At this institution, she developed and co-led parent-child activity groups as well as provided individual parent-child occupation-based treatment. She has presented on the topic of parent-child activity groups at numerous local, national and international conferences, as well as on other topics related to pediatric occupational therapy. In addition to publishing research about pediatric occupational therapy practice, she has also written extensively about child and adolescent psychosocial occupational therapy practice.

Dr. Olson received a Doctor of Philosophy Degree in Occupational Therapy from New York University in 2002. The first 7 chapters of this book were part of her dissertation, *Interactions Among Participants in a Parent-Child Activity Group on a Child Inpatient Unit.*

Dr. Olson is actively involved in the New York State Occupational Therapy Association (NYSOTA) as Westchester District Chairperson and is currently representing NYSOTA in IDEA Partnership activities. She was the co-chair of the NYSOTA Conference at the United Nations (August 2006).

Foreword

It is an awesome responsibility and privilege to introduce this text. This book offers important information about improving occupational therapy services to children with mental health disabilities and their families. I took the opportunity of preparing for this foreword by reflecting on my own childhood. How did I develop the appreciation for activities that are at the core of my professional beliefs about human occupation? Why do I feel so strongly that the core of occupational therapy is embedded in our ability to create interventions that address the whole person, including their mental health needs? Do these core beliefs stem from my childhood?

Reflecting on my childhood with my mother, father, and two brothers brought to mind multiple visual images and memories. Each visual image was framed by an event. While I could remember the event and some details of what happened, my reflections seemed limited by lack of details of what exactly happened. What I do remember is what we did together as a family. My recollections of event memories were collective feelings around a specific event or activity. A camping adventure into the forest of the Colorado Rocky Mountains included camping, cooking, walking trails, and stories around the campfire. The recall ends with going to sleep in a tent or out in the open campground. These were really family centered group activities.

My life experiences reflect the three key important concepts proposed in this text: family-centered, activity groups, and the therapeutic value of activities and occupations. Family-centered intervention is a philosophical construct that recognizes the importance of all members of the family as a group. Family groups exist for the benefit of all mem-

---

[Haworth co-indexing entry note]: "Foreword." Hinojosa, Jim. Co-published simultaneously in *Occupational Therapy in Mental Health* (The Haworth Press, Inc.) Vol. 22, No. 3/4, 2006, pp. xix-xxi; and: *Activity Groups in Family-Centered Treatment: Psychiatric Occupational Therapy Approaches for Parents and Children* (Laurette Olson) The Haworth Press, Inc., 2006, pp. xv-xvii. Single or multiple copies of this article are available for a fee from The Haworth Document Delivery Service [1-800- HAWORTH, 9:00 a.m. - 5:00 p.m. (EST). E-mail address: docdelivery@haworthpress.com].

xv

bers. No one member is more important than any other. The goals of the family groups are to create and support a smooth and efficient operation of the entire family. When the family includes children, the group shifts its focus and functions to ensure that the children have a safe and appropriate environment within which they can develop and grow. But, this shift recognizes that each family member is equally important in the family structure and the occupations of the family's support the integrity of the whole family.

Societies form around groups. Members of groups interact and engage in activities for pleasure, self-mastery, development, or to occupy their time. From these activities, occupations emerge that reflect the culture, beliefs, and values of the societal group. Occupational therapists value the use of activity groups as a therapeutic medium. While the focus of this book is parent and child activity groups within the psychiatric setting, in the real world activities are the foundation upon which family members interact with each other. The importance of these activities should not be minimized.

Family members interact around a wide range of occupations. The scope of these occupations varies based upon the family's culture, economic resources, values and opportunities available. When working with all families, it is essential that therapists use their knowledge and skills to enhance a family's ability to engage in occupation within the context of a family group. This text provides insight into our understanding of the therapeutic uses self in the group situation. Based on her doctoral dissertation, Dr. Olson shares what she learned. This text provides information that can guide our reflections of our own practices. For me, her findings reaffirmed my commitment to the value of appropriate activities as therapeutic media. Most important, it led me to realize that it is not the activity or group themselves that are therapeutic. It is the therapist's theory driven actions that are therapeutic. Simple therapeutic responses and actions can have a profound effect!

Dr. Olson's description of parent-child activity groups highlights a high degree of knowledge and skills that are needed to insure that they are effective. She identifies the multiple skills that therapists must have to create effective interventions. For occupational therapists, Dr. Olson challenges us to use our expertise in therapeutic use of self, group process, and our understanding of family member roles and responsibilities to address mental health concerns of our clients. These fundamental aspects of occupational therapy seem less valued today. This text supports the importance and value of activity groups and the therapeutic use of self. I am confident that each person that reads this text will find ideas that they can apply both to their own life as a therapist, and also to their lives as members of social groups.

Jim Hinojosa, PhD, OT, FAOTA
Professor and Chair
New York University

Preface

In this volume, *Activity Groups in Family-Centered Treatment: Psychiatric Occupational Therapy Approaches for Parents and Children*, I share a qualitative research study that I completed for my dissertation, as well as case studies from my clinical work with psychiatrically hospitalized adolescents and their parents and a young mother diagnosed with depression and her baby. As the reader will learn in the first chapter, I found providing parent-child occupation-based interventions to be the most important services that I offered while working at a psychiatric facility. I came to understand the pain and gap that mental illness can drive into a parent-child relationship. The activities that are most frequently cherished by parents and their typically developing children and also strengthen parent-child bonds–playing a game, cooking together, enjoying conversation over a meal–may be rare, filled with tension or absent in families that include a child or parent with mental illness. In this book, I will explore how parent-child occupation-based interventions may support the capacity of families that include a parent or child with mental illness to participate and find pleasure in the everyday family co-occupations.

Laurette Olson, PhD, OTR/L

[Haworth co-indexing entry note]: "Preface." Olson, Laurette. Co-published simultaneously in *Occupational Therapy in Mental Health* (The Haworth Press, Inc.) Vol. 22, No. 3/4, 2006, p. xxiii; and: *Activity Groups in Family-Centered Treatment: Psychiatric Occupational Therapy Approaches for Parents and Children* (Laurette Olson) The Haworth Press, Inc., 2006, p. xix. Single or multiple copies of this article are available for a fee from The Haworth Document Delivery Service [1-800- HAWORTH, 9:00 a.m. - 5:00 p.m. (EST). E-mail address: docdelivery@haworthpress.com].

Acknowledgements

This work would not have been possible without my opportunity to learn from the many parents and children that I have had the honor to work with over the course of my career. In particular, I offer my deep gratitude to the families and leaders who participated in my qualitative research study about parent-child activity groups. With deep appreciation, I also thank the families who participated in the parent-adolescent group and "Eileen," the young mother with depression and her family whom I had the opportunity to get to know and work with over several years.

I also extend my gratitude to the many professionals with whom I have been fortunate enough to call colleagues. They supported, befriended and mentored me as I learned about working with parents and children. I recognize that I have had outstanding learning opportunities over the course of my career and hope that this work lives up to the expectations of my past colleagues.

The late Dr. Paulina Kernberg was a constant support and mentor to me when I was a young occupational therapist learning about working with children and families in a large teaching hospital filled with many seasoned mental health professionals. I was entranced with her amazing ability to engage even the children most withdrawn from human interaction. She welcomed me into the clinical and academic community of the child and adolescent psychiatric division that she led. She engaged me in a number of interesting and challenging clinical, academic, and research projects that pushed me to see myself differently and led me to develop my work and myself well beyond what I imagined I could do as an occupational therapist.

[Haworth co-indexing entry note]: "Acknowledgements." Olson, Laurette. Co-published simultaneously in *Occupational Therapy in Mental Health* (The Haworth Press, Inc.) Vol. 22, No. 3/4, 2006, pp. xxv-xxvi; and: *Activity Groups in Family-Centered Treatment: Psychiatric Occupational Therapy Approaches for Parents and Children* (Laurette Olson) The Haworth Press, Inc., 2006, pp. xxi-xxii. Single or multiple copies of this article are available for a fee from The Haworth Document Delivery Service [1-800- HAWORTH, 9:00 a.m. - 5:00 p.m. (EST). E-mail address: docdelivery@haworthpress.com].

Barbara Milone, CSW, Colleen Heaney, MS, and Lauren Quintana, RN, have been my co-leaders of parent-child activity group, my supports, sounding boards, and dear friends. Barbara Milone presented a paper with me about parent-adolescent activity groups at a Grand Rounds presentation at a teaching hospital and at a professional conference. That presentation was the basis of the parent-adolescent chapter in this book.

My qualitative research study would not have taken place without the support and guidance of Dr. Jim Hinojosa, the chair of my dissertation committee at New York University. He provided me with the opportunity to pursue doctoral studies through the Maternal Child Health Training Grant that he wrote and directed. Throughout the process of my doctoral coursework, writing my dissertation proposal, completing my research, and struggling through the challenging process of making sense of my data, his support, guidance, insight, and pragmatism kept me focused. I am very grateful for my opportunity to be his student. Dr. Joanne Griffin shared her outstanding ability to think divergently and continually challenged me to think more deeply throughout the process of data analysis. She helped me to think about my data in more ways than I imagined that I could. Dr. Margot Ely's talent as a qualitative researcher is unparalleled. She offered very insightful comments that fostered my staying focused on using strong qualitative methods throughout my research, data analysis, and presentation of my findings. Dr. Mauritizio Zambenedetti was a wonderful advocate and support to me within the hospital system where my research was carried out.

This volume would not have been written without the encouragement, support, and amazing patience of Dr. Mary Donohue and Marie-Louis Blount, AM, OT, FAOTA, the co-editors of *Occupational Therapy in Mental Health.* I appreciate the structure and opportunity to share my ideas about parent child occupation-based intervention.

I could not end my acknowledgements without thanking my family. My parents have been consistently supportive throughout my life and my career. They have always been willing to help in whatever way they could. Along with the rest of my family, they have endured my evolving thinking about parent-child activity interaction which included serving as models for pictures that have accompanied my writings on the topic. I have cherished my opportunity to be the aunt of Mark, Kathryn, Elizabeth, Carolyn and Kevin. They have been my best teachers about childhood and what children need from their adult caregivers. They have had more influence on my work than they will ever understand.

Chapter 1

Introduction

SUMMARY. This chapter provides an overview of this volume as well as a description of the author's experiences working with psychiatrically hospitalized children and their families that led her to develop the framework for parent-child occupation-based group and individual intervention that is described in this publication. doi:10.1300/J004v22n03_01 *[Article copies available for a fee from The Haworth Document Delivery Service: 1-800-HAWORTH. E-mail address: <docdelivery@haworthpress.com> Website: <http://www.HaworthPress.com> © 2006 by The Haworth Press, Inc. All rights reserved.]*

KEYWORDS. Occupational therapy, parent-child activity groups, child psychiatry

In the first seven chapters of this volume, I will describe my experiences as a researcher studying the experiences of a group of parents and their psychiatrically hospitalized children as they participated in a parent-child activity group on a child inpatient unit. In the following two chapters, I will share some of my other experiences adapting my parent-child activity group work for addressing the needs of parents and their psychiatrically hospitalized adolescent offspring and a mother diagnosed

[Haworth co-indexing entry note]: "Introduction." Olson, Laurette. Co-published simultaneously in *Occupational Therapy in Mental Health* (The Haworth Press, Inc.) Vol. 22, No. 3/4, 2006, pp. 1-9; and: *Activity Groups in Family-Centered Treatment: Psychiatric Occupational Therapy Approaches for Parents and Children* (Laurette Olson) The Haworth Press, Inc., 2006, pp. 1-9. Single or multiple copies of this article are available for a fee from The Haworth Document Delivery Service [1-800- HAWORTH, 9:00 a.m. - 5:00 p.m. (EST). E-mail address: docdelivery@haworthpress.com].

with depression and her baby–persons with mental illness within the context of their families that include children.

I began my career as an occupational therapist expecting to provide individual and group services for children. In my second year of practice, I began working as an occupational therapist with children on a child inpatient psychiatric unit. Most of the children were hospitalized because of severe behavior outbursts, including the destruction of property and physical violence or threats toward adults, other children, or themselves. Their relationships with their parents were typically tense; the parents spoke of being overwhelmed and unable to manage their children's behavior prior to the hospitalization. Many of these children and their parents described little or no pleasurable parent-child interaction immediately prior to hospitalization.

On the child inpatient unit, I frequently worked with children who showed little enjoyment or investment in play or activity when they were alone, in groups, or with their parents. They quickly expressed feeling overwhelmed, frustrated, or bored when an activity presented a challenge to them. Over the course of their hospitalization, many of these children developed interests and began to enjoy play and activity on the unit, but their interactions with their parents did not substantially change.

I observed little playful interaction occurring between parents and children on the unit. Children expressed a longing each day for visits from their families. When visiting hours finally came, I observed distant and superficial interaction between some parents and children; others had tense visits that ended in children being reprimanded for misbehavior. It was anticlimactic for some of the children whose needs for positive contact and interaction with their families were not met. The following day, these children again longed for their next visit with their families.

When I spoke to other staff about my observations, I was frequently told that life for these children was not going to change. The sentiment of the staff was that children who had negative relationships with their parents would likely continue to have that type of relationship with them, and that their behavior would most likely deteriorate after discharge from the hospital.

Varied therapeutic approaches were used on the unit to assist families in providing greater structure so that children might be successfully reintegrated into their families. These methods included teaching behavior management techniques to parents and providing family therapy and individual parent counseling. In spite of these efforts, many of the professionals with whom I worked spoke of the strong resistance of these families toward making changes in parent-child interaction. I felt that as an occupational therapist, I could design a group that would complement the work of others and would add a different dimension to what was presently offered to these families.

I developed a parent-child activity group based on the premise that if children's play behavior could change in a positive direction with the staff and other children on the inpatient unit, it could also change with their parents. I believed that an activity group that increased opportunities for positive interaction between parent and child might lessen the degree of negative interaction between some children and parents. A structured play group might change the expectations of both parents and children, and lead to pleasurable interactions. Over time, if families had multiple positive experiences, they might begin to expect pleasure in family activity and thus seek out opportunities for similar parent-child interaction outside of the group.

I based my parent-child activity group organization on what I heard about a similar group that occurred in another hospital, and on my knowledge of group theory (Cartwright & Zander, 1968; Yalom, 1995), occupational therapy theory (Fidler & Fidler, 1978; Reilly, 1974), and parent-child interaction research and theory (Heard, 1981; Lytton, 1980; Murphy, 1962; Murphy & Moriarty, 1976). I organized the parent-child activity group as a multifamily group in which everyday constructional activities, tabletop or gross motor games, or play were used as a concrete means to engage individual family members with each other in a manner that they would likely perceive as pleasurable and positive. Since other families were also present and participating in activities with their own members, there was an opportunity to learn from other families via observation, as well as through interaction. My co-leaders and I adapted activities to limit the impact of children or parents' attentional difficulties, motor planning or coordination deficits in order to support the ability of parents and children to participate in everyday family leisure or activities of daily living that had the potential to draw parents and children closer and to be more in tune with each other. My goal was for children to expect warmth, positive attention and assistance from parents and for parents to expect warmth, cooperation, and compliance from their children.

As I led the parent-child activity group, I observed that some parents appeared to be walking on eggshells, afraid that their children might have a tantrum if they set limits. They seemed to do whatever their children demanded to get through the first groups that they attended. Other parents actively avoided interaction with their children in activity; they appeared angry and ready for trouble between themselves and their children. As they were helped to interact and participate in projects and activities with their children by the leaders and their observations of other families, they seemed to relax and interact with their children with increased pleasure. Some parents took over projects from their children when there was a display of the kind of misbehavior that the parents seemed to expect. As parents and children became comfortable in the group and began to use the support and assistance of the group leaders and other members, the children remained more consistently involved in activity with their parents and the activities were more often child-directed. Children were reprimanded less, and parents and children exhibited more pleasure in their interaction. I observed parents and children smiling at one another and talking about their days as they worked together to complete a project or to play a game. Some parents and children reported that they had not experienced the other in this way before and structured similar activities for their other time together during the week. Over time, parents exhibited more interest in participating in activities with their children on and off the inpatient unit. Some also appeared to develop a more optimistic view of interacting with their children.

In my informal conversations with some parent participants, they told me that they had not expected the experience of a parent-child activity group to be positive or productive. They said that it took a few sessions to be comfortable with the idea. They reported that watching other families participate in activities and listening to them discuss successes, as well as difficulties, were very helpful. Other professionals reported that after this group, some parents and children were more positively engaged with each other at other times on the ward and more open to other forms of therapy.

The following are excerpts from a taped interview with Susan, a mother who participated in parent-child activity group during a late spring and summer in the early 1990's when I was a co-leader of the group. The interview took place midsummer prior to her discharge from the parent-child group. Though her situation was different from that of the other parent participants because Susan was an inpatient on an adult psychiatric unit at the same hospital, she reported feelings about herself as a parent similar to those I heard from other parents who were visiting their hospitalized children. She came to participate in the group because it seemed that she and her children had similar issues and would likely fit comfortably into the group. In the course of our retrospective discussion about her experiences in the parent-child activity group, Susan brought up some reactions to the group process that were similar to what I had heard from other parents who had participated in the group.

Susan's children came to the hospital to participate in the group. Her sons, Tommy and David, were 11- and 7-years-old respectively. All names are pseudonyms.

Susan talked about her feelings about herself:

> I felt inadequate. I'm not really that artistic and so it was important that I be able to think of all of the wonderful ideas and do a good job so that this will show that I'm a really good mom . . . that everything is perfect and that was very hard in the beginning. It seems like that was what I was concentrating on. Even more than interaction with the boys.

Susan shared some thoughts about working with her sons in parent-child group:

> One of the things that were difficult in the beginning that changed was the feeling of walking on eggs with each other. I was afraid I was going to say the wrong thing and I think they were afraid that they would say the wrong thing . . . I remember, in the very beginning, I couldn't think about how to put anything together, because I felt like I had to think of this all on my own and I had to think of the idea and I had to put this together. Later on, as the interaction between us became better and more relaxed, the idea came from all of us. I would throw something out, Tommy would say maybe we could add this, or my other son, David would say, "Mommy, what about this?" By the end of the project, everyone has put in an idea and no matter what it looks like, it's really special, no matter what it is . . . We laughed at some of our projects, but we thought they were pretty terrific because we all helped. One time with the four of us–we still have it at home. We made a house and all of us had a different part. I made the curtains and the bedspreads; my husband made the roof; Tommy helped paint inside; David made our family–with clothespins. We all had a pillow. We all had a bed. It was the four of us and it was very special because we did it together.

> I did get relaxed. You know, it's not just playing with them. It's learning, learning how to sit down and learn how to enjoy being together and I've always had a hard time with that because I always

thought things had to be perfect. Or, you know, I shouldn't be a mother if anything not going to be perfect, but that's not true. . . If the project came out perfect that would show that I'm doing what I'm supposed to be doing. It was not what I wanted and it was not what they wanted. . .

Susan shared her thoughts about being in a group with other families:

I learned a lot by watching and hearing what was going on with other people and mostly I think as far as that goes, that I learned that I was not the only one having a difficult time. I always thought that I was one of very few people that had a hard time with knowing how to sit down with my kids and that was hard. I didn't think I was going to learn much of that, but I did. I'm not the only parent who has a hard time and it's not like you have to have a hard time for the rest of your life. You can work on it. . .

The literature that I read at the time of initiating my first parent-child activity group and the subsequent literature that I have read support engaging families as I have done through group or individual parent-child activity intervention. Unfortunately, psychiatric services are often splintered into services for children and services for the adults in their lives. In many settings, only a small portion of resources is directed toward engaging family members with each other. Consistent with this, many occupational therapists typically see their roles as supporting the function of individual family members and consulting with family members as a supplement to reinforce intervention goals in children's everyday lives outside of therapy. Over eight years of leading and supervising parent-child activity groups as an occupational therapist at a psychiatric facility, I came to believe that my most profound influence on my clients was through my work engaging parents and children in the actual doing of meaningful play and leisure activities. For the parents and children with mental illness that I will describe in this book, it was critical that parents were key figures in their children's occupation-based treatment and experienced themselves as competent in supporting their children's successful participation in everyday play and leisure activities. Many of these parents and children struggled with each other in their co-occupations for years prior to their children's hospitalization and had come to believe that it is not possible to succeed at and enjoy co-occupations. Consultation was not enough in supporting improved family function in the interest of child development. Actual experience over time may positively shift parents' beliefs about their skills as parents, children's beliefs that their parents will be able to support them in their activities and children's capacity to be cooperative and engage with parents in joint activity.

As my work and that of my colleagues whom I engaged as co-leaders in the parent-child activity group became an important part of the psychiatric services offered on the child inpatient unit, my colleagues and I were asked to work with other groups of patients at the hospital. I developed and co-led a parent-adolescent activity group on the adolescent inpatient unit, a parent-child activity group for preschool children at risk for developing behavior disorders at a local preschool (Olson, Heaney, & Soppas, 1989), and began providing individual and group parent-child intervention for parents hospitalized with mental illness and their children.

Within this volume, I will first share my research on parent child activity group intervention on a child inpatient psychiatric unit. In Chapter 2, I will present the theory and research literature that describes the nature of the interaction between parents and children with emotional disorders. I will then present professional writings about the issues arising between parents and children around a child's psychiatric hospitalization and the nature of family involvement in psychiatric settings. Jumping off from this literature, I will describe then the framework that I developed for parent-child activity groups and for individual parent-child occupational therapy intervention.

In Chapter 3, I introduce readers to some of the families who participated in the parent-child activity group that I studied. By providing readers with a rich description of the challenges faced by some of the families that I've met in a parent-child activity group, as well as the strengths that these families exhibited, I hope to engage them thinking more deeply about whom the members of these families are. Readers may find that something that resonates with their own experiences with parents and children with mental illness.

I present my framework for parent-child activity groups in Chapter 4. In addition, I developed snapshots of a parent-child activity group to help readers visualize the parent-child activity group that I studied for my dissertation research. In Chapter 5, readers learn about my research methods and some of the results of my qualitative study including what I came to understand about what families appeared to gain through their participation in parent-child group. I explore the barriers that seemed to interfere with parents and children exploring how to engage in the co-occupation of parent-child play and leisure activity in the parent-child activity group that I studied, as well as my reflections on how to remove those barriers in similar parent-child activity groups. My research is a first step in examining what may happen in such a group and what clinicians can learn from those experiences to better provide services that support families that include a child with mental illness in having positive experiences in their co-occupations. Therefore in Chapter 7, I reconsider my thinking about parent-child activity groups and how my framework might be refined.

In Chapter 8, I share some of my clinical experiences leading a parent-adolescent activity group on an adolescent inpatient unit. I present case descriptions developed from logs that my co-leaders and I wrote as we worked with the families described and refined our group approach. I found that leading groups for adolescents and their parents required adapting the approach that I used for school age children and their parents. My experience was that in spite of adolescents' increasing independence from their parents, that the adolescents that I met desired and needed to have positive interactions and relationships with their parents. This is consistent with the literature about renegotiating the parent-child relationship in adolescence.

I will share my experiences providing parent-child intervention as an occupational therapist for a young woman hospitalized for depression, her baby, and her husband in Chapter 9. I worked with this family during this woman's short term hospitalization and then continued to work with her and her family within their home environment over the following 2 1/2 years. This chapter is based upon detailed logs written as I worked with this family.

In the final chapter of this volume, Chapter 10, I will share my closing thoughts about what I have learned through my clinical experiences and research about helping parents and children more fully and positively participate in their co-occupations. I became interested and involved in studying and providing services in this area of psychosocial rehabilitation because I saw striking deficits in the co-occupations of the families that I met. No services met the needs that I observed. The occupational therapy profession could potentially meet this critical consumer need while also complementing the work done by other mental health professionals. It is important that occupational therapists increase their study of interventions to support parents and children in developing optimal interaction patterns for occupational health and development of all family members in spite of mental illness and in support of mental health.

REFERENCES

Cartwright, D., & Zander, A. (Eds.). (1968). *Group dynamics: Research and theory* (3rd Ed.). New York: Harper & Row.

Fidler, G. S., & Fidler, J. W. (1978). Doing and becoming: Purposeful action and self-actualization. *American Journal of Occupational Therapy, 32,* 305-310.

Heard, D. H. (1981). From object relations to attachment theory: A basis for family therapy. *British Journal of Medical Psychology, 51,* 67-76.

Lytton, H. (1980). *Attachment in parent-child interaction.* New York: Plenum Press.

Murphy, L. (1962). *The widening world of childhood.* New York: Basic Books.

Murphy, L., & Moriarty, A. (1976). *Vulnerability, coping, and growth from infancy to adolescence.* New Haven, CT: Yale University Press.

Reilly, M. (Ed.). (1974). *Play as exploratory learning.* Beverly Hills, CA: Sage.

Yalom, I. D. (1995). *The Theory and Practice of Group Psychotherapy* (4th Ed.). NY: Basic Books.

doi:10.1300/J004v22n03_01

Chapter 2

What Do We Know About the Daily Interactions Between Children with Mental Illness and Their Parents?

SUMMARY. This chapter is a literature review that explores the nature of interaction between parents and children with emotional disorders, issues between parents and professionals when children are psychiatrically hospitalized, and the nature of parent involvement in child psychiatric settings. doi:10.1300/J004v22n03_02 *[Article copies available for a fee from The Haworth Document Delivery Service: 1-800-HAWORTH. E-mail address: <docdelivery@haworthpress.com> Website: <http://www.HaworthPress.com> © 2006 by The Haworth Press, Inc. All rights reserved.]*

KEYWORDS. Children with mental illness, parent participation, child psychiatric treatment

This literature review is divided into four sections central to my parent-child activity group research described in this volume. I first review

---

[Haworth co-indexing entry note]: "What Do We Know About the Daily Interactions Between Children with Mental Illness and Their Parents?" Olson, Laurette. Co-published simultaneously in *Occupational Therapy in Mental Health* (The Haworth Press, Inc.) Vol. 22, No. 3/4, 2006, pp. 11-22; and: *Activity Groups in Family-Centered Treatment: Psychiatric Occupational Therapy Approaches for Parents and Children* (Laurette Olson) The Haworth Press, Inc., 2006, pp. 11-22. Single or multiple copies of this article are available for a fee from The Haworth Document Delivery Service [1-800- HAWORTH, 9:00 a.m. - 5:00 p.m. (EST). E-mail address: docdelivery@haworthpress.com].

Available online at http://otmh.haworthpress.com
© 2006 by The Haworth Press, Inc. All rights reserved.
doi:10.1300/J004v22n03_02

how the interactions between parents and their emotionally disturbed children have been described. I then discuss the issues and concerns that arise between parents and professionals when children are psychiatrically hospitalized. In the third section, I review the reported ways that families of children who have been psychiatrically hospitalized or placed in a psychiatric residential facility have been helped to interact with their children at the institutions, and finally I discuss the theories that served as a basis for the development of the parent-child activity group that was studied.

NATURE OF INTERACTION BETWEEN PARENTS AND CHILDREN WITH EMOTIONAL DISORDERS

Studies have shown that the nature of parent-child interaction is more problematic in families where a child is described as having oppositional defiant disorder, conduct disorder, or depression, than in families where children are adequately functioning (Crowell, Feldman & Ginsberg, 1988; Dadds, Sanders, Morrison & Rebgetz, 1992; Dumas, 1996; Field et al., 1987; Johnston, 1996). Aversive interchanges between mothers and children have been a strong finding in some studies that attempted to differentiate children who receive psychiatric services from those who do not (Dadds et al., 1992; Dumas & LaFreniere, 1993; Dumas, 1996; Sanders, Dadds, & Bor, 1989).

There is debate on whether levels of positive behavior that occur between parents and children are different in families that include children with psychiatric diagnoses as opposed to families that do not. Dadds et al. (1992) stated that there is no difference. They studied families' interactions by filming a group of families eating dinner as a family unit one time. The novelty of the camera and the presence of observers in the homes on a single occasion likely changed the typical behavior of the participants. Families may have consciously tried to present their best behavior to the researchers. In other studies, levels of positive interaction differed between families in which a child exhibited high levels of aggressive or anxious behavior from families in which a child did not exhibit problem behavior (Dumas et al., 1992; Dumas & LaFreniere, 1993; Dumas, 1996; Pettit & Bates, 1989).

Families with disruptive children exhibited low levels of positive interaction and compliance coupled with high levels of aggression between mothers and children. In the 1996 study, Dumas' methodology included six unstructured home observations for one hour each time over a period of two to three weeks. With more persistent observations over a period of time, this researcher more likely had the opportunity to observe more typical parent-child interaction than the one-time observation by Dadd et al. (1992).

In a 1984 review article, Mash reported that mothers of problem children react less favorably even when their children initiated appropriate interaction. He concluded that positive behavior occurring in the context of a negative relationship may not be perceived as positive. Other studies have noted the noncontingent nature of mothers' responses to their children with behavior problems (Dumas, LaFreniere, Beaudin, & Verlaan, 1992; Dumas, LaFreniere, & Serketich, 1995; Field et al., 1987; Snyder, 1977). A child's positive behavior might receive either a negative or positive parental response.

Parents of children who are psychiatrically hospitalized reported that they have negative expectations of their children (Preston, 1990). Preston proposed that these negative expectations might be a link to understanding the children's continued negative behavior and the conflict between parent and child. Parents who expect that their children will misbehave may begin interactions with these children in defensive ways. They may seek control or fear loss of control instead of engaging their child in relaxed everyday interactions. In kind, children may respond with resistance to the attempts to control them. To carry out his study, Preston (1990) interviewed the parents of 76 children who were psychiatrically hospitalized. In these interviews, parents were asked about past or hypothetical interactions with their children; they were not asked about current interactions. This may increase the possibility that parents might distort their recollection of their interactions with their children. Preston (1990) stated that direct observations of parent-child interaction and concurrent interviewing might be a more effective way to understand parents' perceptions of their children.

In examining family interaction in families that included a child labeled as delinquent, Alexander, Barton, Waldron, and Mas (1989) found that when a researcher facilitated a positive focus in family verbal interaction, members were less accusatory of each other than they were when families discussed problem behaviors. They stated that the positive effect on family interaction did not last after the families were allowed to interact in typical negative ways, but they suggested that repeated opportunities to interact in a positive context might lead to a lasting change in how families interact. Findings from their study suggest that it may be as important or more important to focus on positive interactions as opposed to just addressing negative interactions in therapy.

Fostering positive interaction between parents and their children who are psychiatrically hospitalized within a structured activity group over time may help to lessen the negative views that parents might have of their children. This may lead to increased positive behavior by the children in response to the positive attention that they receive from their parents. Learning about how parents and their psychiatrically hospitalized children feel about their participation in a parent-child activity group may lead to further elaboration and refinement of this intervention method.

ISSUES BETWEEN PARENTS AND PROFESSIONALS WHEN CHILDREN ARE PSYCHIATRICALLY HOSPITALIZED

Throughout the literature, it is reported that parents feel blamed by professionals and excluded in overt and covert ways from participation in their children's treatment by professionals (Collins, Collins, Botyrius-Maier, & MacIntosh-Daeschler, 1994; Harper & Geraty, 1986; Petr & Barney, 1993; Whittaker, 1981). Blaming leads to disempowerment and alienation of parents who likely already feel guilt about their inability to manage their child. Parents are less likely to engage in their children's therapy when they feel judged. To empower parents, many theorists feel that environments need to be structured so that parents feel competent in their interactions with their children and valued as allies in their children's treatment by staff (Collins & Collins, 1990; Palmer, Harper & Rivinus, 1983; Street & Treacher, 1986; Whittaker, 1981).

Professionals may view the experience of children within their families prior to psychiatric hospitalization very differently from the parents. For many of these children, their relationship with their parents has deteriorated to the point that neither parent nor child seems to derive pleasure or benefit from their interaction. Parents may not support, help, or monitor their children's behavior in everyday activities because they experience their children as unresponsive and themselves as ineffective. This might be described as parents' rejecting their children; Street and Treacher (1986) suggest that something more complex is occurring and describe the process as "developmental closure." Over time, these parents and children may have gradually lost their ability to manage their interactions so that the children can be parented successfully. Parents may not experience competence in their role and neither they nor the children may derive any sense of security, satisfaction, and pleasure from their daily interaction. Street and Treacher (1986) suggest that professionals need to reframe how they look at what happens between parents and their children prior to the children's placement in a psychiatric facility. The explanation of the situation must facilitate intervention, and it cannot if the parents feel blame and alienation. The end goal of most child psychiatric treatment is to assist parents to manage their children's mental illness so that they can physically and emotionally support their children and enable them to become productive adults. The hospitalization should therefore be a time to change their interactions from negative to positive, not a cause of further dislocation.

Another view about what may be happening between parents and professionals when children are psychiatrically hospitalized is a phenomenon labeled an "adoption process" (Palmer, Harper, & Rivinus, 1983). As psychiatric staff develops close relationships with the children while not simultaneously developing close relationships with the children's parents, they may begin to see the children's problems as external to the children. They then begin to protect the children from parents who may be perceived as the cause of the problem and exclude the parents from treatment planning. In reaction to their own feelings of guilt and after observing that their children are behaving better in the hospital and are being well cared for, parents may collude with staff by withdrawing from the unit and their children. Palmer, Harper, and Rivinus (1983) see this as a maladaptive solution, even though children may be well cared for and parents get relief from having to deal with their children's problematic behavior. Parents are not aided in learning how to manage their children's behavior, to provide for their children's needs, or to enjoy interacting with their children. Children may be caught between two sets of caregivers who are at odds, and pleasing one set of caregivers may lead to the feeling that they are betraying the other set. In this scenario, nothing happens that will affect the children's everyday life after hospitalization. When children are discharged, symptomatic behaviors return and parents have not learned how to handle those behaviors.

The literature strongly suggests that it is insufficient to help children adapt to institutions. When the staff of a psychiatric facility takes over the complete management and treatment of the children in their care, they may inadvertently foster the children's development away from their families, making it less likely that they can be reintegrated into their family's everyday life (Brown, 1991; Palmer, Harper, & Rivinus, 1983; Street & Treacher, 1986). Parents may feel a sense of failure and inadequacy when they simply visit their children at a psychiatric facility. Watching staff manage their children effectively may be counter-therapeutic (Brown, 1991; Palmer, Harper & Rivinus, 1983). Parents may withdraw and experience their influence and connections with their children lessening while observing professionals develop increased influence and strong ties with their children.

In residential programs, research shows that children's behavior does change positively, but upon discharge into families that have not changed, the children's old behaviors reappear. The mission of these institutions is to prepare children for a productive life outside of an institution. Children cannot truly adapt to community life outside of an institution unless their families also change (Finkelstein, 1974).

NATURE OF PARENT INVOLVEMENT IN CHILD PSYCHIATRIC SETTINGS

Throughout the literature, there is strong advocacy for engaging parents and collaborating with them in the psychiatric treatment of their children because parents are their children's long-term caregivers (Berlin, 1978; Brown, 1991; Finkelstein, 1974; Preminger-Dreier & Gordon-Lewis, 1991; Whittaker, 1974; Woolston, 1989). The degree of family involvement has been considered an important prognostic indicator for children with psychiatric illness (Blotcky, Dimperio, & Gossett, 1984; Finkelstein, 1974; Gossett, 1988).

Finkelstein (1974), Harper and Geraty (1986), and Whittaker (1981) stated that parents should be a part of pleasurable unit activities in order to see that adults and children can have fun together; this is essential for reuniting parent and child. Carlo (1985) saw the residential living space of children as an ideal place for parents to learn parenting skills with the support of the staff. Brown (1991) suggested that parents need to be offered more control over their children and a complementary role with staff. Structured visits where parents are supported and helped to positively engage with their children may increase parents' sense of competence, as well as their interest in interacting with their children. Neither Brown (1991), Harper and Geraty (1986), Whittaker (1981), nor Finkelstein (1974) described a structure in which to facilitate this positive parent-child interaction at residential or inpatient facilities.

Berlin (1978) proposed that inpatient staff should always be involved with families during visiting hours so that they can assist parents in engaging their children in appropriate developmental activities. They also should be available to help parents to learn how to encourage their children's best performance. He stated that if parents first learn to effectively engage their children in the hospital setting, they will be more likely to do so at home. Berlin did not carry out any studies to test his theory. Likewise, Greenfield and Senecal (1995) and Olson (1999, 2001) recommended engaging parents in mutual activity with their children and guiding parents in positively and effectively assisting their children. They recommend a multifamily group format where families can support and assist each other in the process of change. Like Berlin, they did not discuss any research that tested their approaches.

Carlo (1993) studied methods of parental involvement in the residential treatment of their children. The independent variables were the particular method of engaging parents (experiential, didactic or both); the dependent variables were a decrease of inappropriate child behavior, movement toward family reunification, and a measure of parental satisfaction with the children's behavior. There were 11 families in the experiential group and 10 families each in the other two groups. The group that received both didactic and experiential opportunities exhibited the greatest positive changes on the dependent variables. The group that received experiential opportunities showed less progress than the group that received didactic instruction alone. Group sizes were small. The members of each group varied significantly; a single parent headed some families, others by the children's biological parents or stepparents. A few families had more than one child in care. Experiential opportunities were described as inviting parents to unit activities with their children such as field trips or birthday parties. Staff was not trained to engage parents with their children. There was no description of how parents were included and whether they were guided in activity with their children. Parents were not provided with a forum so that they could be oriented to experience participating in unit activities with their children or to process what occurred afterwards. While the experience of including parents on the psychiatric unit is reported to have been positive for both parents and children, the opportunity to observe and to use the experience to engage parents with their children with emotional disturbances in new ways was not maximized.

The literature discussed thus far focused on individual parents and children or individual parent-child dyads. Another approach, multiple family group therapy, makes explicit use of the presence of multiple families for therapeutic purposes. The group leaders' primary focus is the overall group process as opposed to the interaction among the members of each family.

Multiple family group therapy has been shown to be an effective technique with adults who were inpatients or outpatients at psychiatric facilities (Brennan, 1995; Laqueur, 1976; McFarlane, Lukas, Link, & Dushay, 1995). This group method as defined by Laqueur (1976) is a verbal group that typically includes approximately four to five families and two co-therapists. It is based on general systems theory that analyzes the input, processing, output, and feedback loops in a system. It is expected that as one person in a system changes, all other persons within the system are affected. In multiple family group therapy, families help each other discover maladaptive behaviors in their family systems. They listen to each other describe family difficulties, question one another to better understand the difficulties, and then offer feedback. Group members change their perspectives on their own family issues as they listen to the stories of other families and receive feedback on the issues that they share. According to the theory of multiple family group therapy, if one person in one family changes, all of the other group participants are affected.

Multiple family group therapy is considered more effective and efficient than individual family approaches because families can learn by observing or identifying with other families. In addition, therapist cues that are successfully used by one family often spread to other families. McFarlane, Link, Dushay, and Marchal (1995) found that multiple family group therapy extended remissions of psychiatric illness and enhanced functioning more effectively than did single family treatments. Laqueur (1976) reported that he treated approximately 1,500 patients with this method. He reported that families exhibited increased mutual liking, respect, acceptance of shortcomings as well as the ability to use family strengths to enjoy day-to-day living. Some clinicians have applied this method to work with children. Wattie (1994) described such a group, but did not attempt to measure change in families.

Greenspoon (1986) described integrating concepts of multiple family group therapy with art therapy methods. Her approach differed from DeSalvatore and Rosenman (1986), Greenfield and Senecal (1995), and Olson (2001) in that she was not attempting to engage families in a typical play activity that might be generalized. She used art psychodynamically; she wanted to diagnose family dynamics and then used art activity as an alternate method of communication within the family and with other families.

No research was found that studied whether parents and their psychiatrically hospitalized children are helped to lessen cycles of negative interactions and to increase their amount of positive interaction in activity through multifamily activity groups. Further, no research was found that has documented persistent credible and trustworthy observation of parents and their psychiatrically hospitalized children while they participate in a parent-child activity group. In Chapter 5, I will describe my qualitative research methods that I used to persistently observe parents and their psychiatrically hospitalized children as they participated in a parent-child group and interviewed both parents and children about their experiences.

REFERENCES

Alexander, J. F., Waldron, H. B., Barton, C., & Mas, C. H. (1989). The minimizing of blaming attributions and behaviors in delinquent families. *Journal of Consulting and Clinical Psychology, 57*, 19-24.

Arend, R., Gore, F. L., & Sroufe, L. A. (1979). Continuity of individual adaptation from infancy to kindergarten. A predictive study of ego resiliency and curiosity in preschoolers. *Child Development, 50*, 950-957.

Bates, J. E. (1976). Effects of children's nonverbal behavior upon adults. *Child Development, 47*, 1079-1088.

Berlin, I. N. (1978). Developmental issues in the psychiatric hospitalization of children. *American Journal of Psychiatry, 135*, 1044-1048.

Blotcky, M. J., Dimperio, T. L., & Gossett, J. T. (1984). Follow-up of children treated in psychiatric hospitals. *American Journal of Psychiatry, 141*, 1499-1507.

Brennan, J. W. (1995). A short-term psychoeducational multiple-family group for bipolar patients and their families. *Social Work, 40*, 737-743.

Brown, J. E. (1991). Family involvement in the residential treatment of children: A systemic perspective. *Australian and New Zealand Journal of Family Therapy, 12(1)*, 17-22.

Bugental, D. B., Caporael, L., & Shennum, W. A. (1980). Experimentally produced child uncontrollability: Effects on the potency of adult communication patterns. *Child Development, 51*, 520-528.

Carlo, P. (1985). The children's residential treatment center as a living laboratory for family members: A review of the literature and its implications for practice. *Child Care Quarterly, 14(3)*, 156-170.

Carlo, P. (1993). Parent education vs. parent involvement: Which type of efforts work best to reunify families? *Journal of Social Service Research, 17*, 135-151.

Chapman, M. (1981). Isolating casual effects through experimental changes in parent-child interaction. *Journal of Abnormal Child Psychology, 9*, 321-327.

Collins, B. G., & Collins, T. M. (1990). Parent-professional relationships in the treatment of seriously emotionally disturbed children and adolescents. *Social Work, 35*, 522-527.

Collins, B. G., Collins, T. M., Botyrius-Maier, G., & MacIntosh-Daeschler, S. (1994). Mental health professionals' perceptions of parent-professional collaboration. *Journal of Mental Health Counseling, 16*, 261-274.

Cook, W. L., Kenny, D. A., & Goldstein, M. J. (1991). Parental affective style risk and the family system: A social relations model analysis. *Journal of Abnormal Psychology*, *100*, 492-501.

Crowell, J. A., Feldman, S. S., & Ginsberg, N. (1988). Assessment of mother-child interaction in preschoolers with behavior problems. *Journal of the Academy of Child and Adolescent Psychiatry*, *27*, 303-311.

Dadds, M. R., Sanders, M. R., Morrison, M., & Rebgetz, M. (1992). Childhood depression and conduct disorder II: An analysis of family interaction patterns in the home. *Journal of Abnormal Psychology*, *101*, 505-513.

Dumas, J. E., & LaFreniere, P. J. (1993). Mother-child relationships as sources of support or stress: A comparison of competent, average, aggressive, and anxious dyads. *Child Development*, *64*, 1732-1754.

Dumas, J. E., LaFreniere, P. J., Beaudin, L., & Verlaan, P. (1992). Mother-child interactions in competent and aggressive dyads: Implications of relationship stress for behaviour therapy with families. *New Zealand Journal of Psychology*, *21*, 3-13.

Dumas, J. E., LaFreniere, P. J., & Serketich, W. J. (1995). Balance of power: A transactional analysis of control in mother-child dyads involving socially competent, aggressive, and anxious children. *Journal of Abnormal Psychology*, *104*, 104-113.

Dumas, J. E. (1996). Why was this child referred? Interaction correlates of referral status in families of children with disruptive behavior problems. *Journal of Clinical Child Psychology*, *25*, 106-115.

Field, T. M., Sandberg, D., Goldstein, S., Garcia, R., Vega-Lahr, N., Porter, K., & Dowling, M. (1987). Play interactions and interviews of depressed and conduct disorder children and their mothers. *Child Psychiatry and Human Development*, *17*, 213-234.

Finkelstein, N. E. (1974). Family participation in residential treatment. *Child Welfare*, *53*, 570-576.

Gossett, J. T. (1988). Treatment evaluation. In J. G. Looney (Ed.), *Chronic mental illness in children and adolescents* (pp. 193-209). Washington D.C.: American Psychiatric Association Press.

Greene, R. W., & Doyle, A. E. (1999). Toward a transactional conceptualization of oppositional defiant disorder: Implications for assessment and treatment. *Clinical Child and Family Psychology Review*, *2*, 129-148.

Greenfield, B. J., & Senecal, J. (1995). Recreational multifamily therapy for troubled children. *American Journal of Orthopsychiatry*, *65*, 434-439.

Greenspoon, D. B. (1986). Multiple-family group art therapy. *Art Therapy*, *1*, 53-60.

Harper, G., & Geraty, R. (1986). Hospital and residential treatment. In A. J. Solnit, D. J. Cohen, & J. E. Schowalter (Eds.), *Child psychiatry* (Vol. 6, pp. 477-496). NY: Basic Books, Inc.

Johnston, C. (1996). Parent characteristics and parent-child interactions in families of nonproblem children and ADHD children with higher and lower levels of oppositional-defiant behavior. *Journal of Abnormal Child Psychology*, *24*, 85-104.

Laqueur, H. (1976). Multiple family therapy. In P. J. Guerin (Ed.), *Family therapy: Theory and practice* (pp. 405-415). New York: John Wiley & Sons.

Lieberman, A. F. (1977). Preschoolers' competence with a peer: Influence of attachment and social experience. *Child Development, 48,* 1277-1287.

Lytton, H. (1980). *Attachment in parent-child interaction.* New York: Plenum Press.

Mash, E. J. (1984). Families with problem children [Children in families under stress]. *New Directions for Child Development, 24,* 65-82.

Matas, L., Arend, R., & Sroufe, L. A. (1978). Continuity of adaptation in the second year: The relationship of the quality of attachment and later competence. *Child Development, 49,* 547-556.

McFarlane, W., Link, B., Dushay, R., & Marchal, J. (1995). Psychoeducational multiple family groups: Four year relapse outcome in schizophrenia. *Family Process, 34,* 127-144.

McFarlane, W., Lukas, E., Link, B., & Dushay, R. (1995). Multiple family groups and psychoeducation in the treatment of schizophrenics. *Archives of General Psychiatry, 52,* 679-687.

Olson, L. (1999). Psychosocial frame of reference. In P. Kramer & J. Hinojosa (Eds.), *Frames of reference for pediatric occupational therapy* (2nd Ed., pp. 323-375). Baltimore, MD: Williams and Wilkins.

Olson, L. (2001). Child psychiatry in the USA. In L. Lougher (Ed.), *Occupational Therapy for Child and Adolescent Mental Health* (pp. 173-191). Edinburgh: Churchill Livingstone.

Palmer, A. J., Harper, G., & Rivinus, T. M. (1983). The "adoption process" in the inpatient treatment of children and adolescents. *Journal of the American Academy of Child and Adolescent Psychiatry, 22,* 286-293.

Petr, C. G., & Barney, D. D. (1993). Reasonable efforts for children with disabilities: The parents' perspective. *Social Work, 38,* 247-254.

Pettit, G. S., & Bates, J. E. (1989). Family interaction patterns and children's behavior problems from infancy to 4 years. *Developmental Psychology, 25,* 413-420.

Preminger-Dreier, M. & Gordon-Lewis, M. (1991). Support and psychoeducation for parents of hospitalized mentally ill children. *Health and Social Work, 16,* 11-18.

Preston, T. (1990). Parents' perceptions of behavior in disturbed children: A study of attributions, affect, and expectancies. (Doctoral dissertation, Vanderbilt University, 1990). *Dissertation Abstracts International, 51,* (5-B) 2632.

Sanders, M. R., Dadds, M. R., & Bor, W. (1989). Contextual analysis of child oppositional and maternal aversive behaviors in families of conduct-disordered and nonproblem children. *Journal of Clinical Child Psychology, 18,* 72-83.

Snyder, J. J. (1977). Reinforcement analysis of interaction in problem and nonproblem families. *Journal of Abnormal Psychology, 86,* 528-535.

Street, E., & Treacher, A. (1986). Developmental closure: A family systems approach to separation in residential care. *Maladjustment and Therapeutic Education, 4(2),* 42-47.

Waters, E., Wittman, J., & Sroufe, L. A. (1979). Attachment, positive affect and competence in the peer group: Two studies in construct validation. *Child Development, 50,* 821-829.

Wattie, M. (1994). Multiple group family therapy. *Journal of Child and Youth Care, 9(4),* 31-38.

Whittaker, J. K. (1981). Family involvement in residential treatment: A support system for parents. In A.N. Maluccio & P.A. Sinanoglu (Eds.), *The Challenge of Partnership, Working with Parents of Children in Foster Care* (pp. 67-87). NY: Child Welfare League of America.

Woolston, J. L. (1989). Transactional risk model for short and intermediate term psychiatric inpatient treatment of children. *Journal of the American Academy of Child and Adolescent Psychiatry, 28,* 38-41.

doi:10.1300/J004v22n03_02

Chapter 3

Introducing Parents and Children Participating in One Parent-Child Group on a Child Inpatient Psychiatric Unit

SUMMARY. The parents and children who participated in the qualitative research study of a parent-child activity group that the author completed for her dissertation are introduced through narratives. Their stories were compiled through formal and informal interviews throughout their participation in the parent-child activity group studied. doi:10.1300/J004v22n03_03 *[Article copies available for a fee from The Haworth Document Delivery Service: 1-800-HAWORTH. E-mail address: <docdelivery@haworthpress.com> Website: <http://www.HaworthPress.com> © 2006 by The Haworth Press, Inc. All rights reserved.]*

KEYWORDS. Children with mental illness, parents, narratives

In this chapter, I will describe the children and parents whom I studied when I examined the parent-child activity group at one child psychiatric inpatient unit. In this way, the readers might have a better understanding of some of the children who might be psychiatrically hospitalized.

[Haworth co-indexing entry note]: "Introducing Parents and Children Participating in One Parent-Child Group on a Child Inpatient Psychiatric Unit." Olson, Laurette. Co-published simultaneously in *Occupational Therapy in Mental Health* (The Haworth Press, Inc.) Vol. 22, No. 3/4, 2006, pp. 23-31; and: *Activity Groups in Family-Centered Treatment: Psychiatric Occupational Therapy Approaches for Parents and Children* (Laurette Olson) The Haworth Press, Inc., 2006, pp. 23-31. Single or multiple copies of this article are available for a fee from The Haworth Document Delivery Service [1-800- HAWORTH, 9:00 a.m. - 5:00 p.m. (EST). E-mail address: docdelivery@haworthpress.com].

I developed the parent-child activity group at Green Hills Hospital to meet the needs of children who are part of a family, but who are not living with their families because they are psychiatrically hospitalized. At Green Hills, children may spend time with their parents for two one-hour visits each day. A few parents visit daily; some visit three times a week or less. As the person who developed the group for this particular unit, I believe that the children needed an opportunity to have more playful interactions with their parents than they would ordinarily experience by visiting on the child inpatient unit. The environment on the unit is not structured to engage children with their parents in activity, and often the children are torn between visiting with their parents and playing with other children. Children and parents need a forum in which to re-approach each other in a positive activity and to practice new ways of interacting with each other.

Conversely, the staff of the child inpatient unit needs an alternative method to observe the unique parent-child interactional styles of each family so that staff can provide meaningful support and interventions for them. From this perspective, the children are the key participants and the fulcrum for the group. The primary focus of the interactions of the group leaders and parents is the behavior or needs of the children.

All of the children who were participants in my study were hospitalized because their behavior could not be managed at home. Many were physically aggressive with their parents, siblings, and/or classmates to the degree that the potential for serious physical harm to others was a major concern. Some also threatened or attempted to hurt themselves. Common diagnoses included Attention Deficit Disorder, Depression, Conduct Disorder, and Oppositional Defiant Disorder. A few were diagnosed as having psychotic disorders, Pervasive Developmental Disorder, or obsessive-compulsive disorder. Ten of the 13 children that I came to know best were hospitalized more than once. Five were hospitalized more than once during the time of my study. Each of these five was discharged home after a very short hospitalization. Some went back to the same school program while others were sent to different schools. Four of the five had significant family distress with the child exhibiting very aggressive behavior before the first hospitalization. Out of control aggressive behavior brought all but one back to the hospital within two months. All four were placed outside of the home after their second or third hospitalization. These families re-entered the parent-child group at the time of each hospitalization.

Sam, a 10-year-old boy, was first hospitalized because he hit his mother and became so violent at home that his sister had to call for the police. Sam was discharged two weeks later and was referred to outpatient psychotherapy. A few weeks later, Sam returned to the hospital. On the day before he was re-hospitalized, he left home on a cold fall day wearing just a tee shirt and his underwear; he didn't return for two hours. When his mother asked where he went, Sam said that he didn't know; he couldn't remember. Sam told a psychiatrist that he was hearing voices that were telling him to do things. Sam was discharged home again, but returned once more within two months. This time, he was hitting his mother again and also tried to poison one of his sisters.

Jason. At the age of 10, Jason is psychiatrically hospitalized for the third time. This time he threatened a classmate with a razor after a minor disagreement and was found to be carrying a box cutter to school that he said was for his own protection. He was hospitalized a few months ago after he threatened to set another child on fire. At home, Jason threatened to kill his mother and chased her around the house with a butter knife. The only plan for Jason at the end of his last hospitalization was to send him to a different school. All of the paperwork required for Jason to begin classes had not been fully processed by the time he left Green Hills. Jason's father will be in jail for at least another seven to ten years. His mother's current boyfriend is an ex-convict with whom she has a stormy relationship. Jason's mother says that she has had it with Jason and wants him to go to residential care or to foster care.

Carlos. Mr. and Mrs. Mendez expressed a high degree of concern about taking Carlos, their nine-year-old son, home after a three-week hospitalization. They said that Carlos was still exhibiting a great deal of aggressive behavior in the hospital and would be aggressive with his half-sisters at home. They felt that their time would again be spent keeping their daughters safe from Carlos. Carlos was discharged to a day treatment facility at the hospital and readmitted to the inpatient unit within two weeks. His first comment to me was, "My father hit me with a belt and he's probably going to go to jail." He said this in a matter of fact manner, making eye contact. He didn't seem upset. He pointed to a slightly bruised, but significantly raised area of skin on his thigh.

All but two of the child participants were hospitalized for two months or less. Most were hospitalized for less than one month. The children that I studied in depth were hospitalized at least one month. Twelve out of the 13 children who I came to know best were boys. I observed five girls, but they were hospitalized for shorter periods of time or they only attended the parent-child group one time during my observations.

FAMILIES IN SHARPER FOCUS

Through the use of narratives, the perspectives of four children and their primary caregivers will be described, focusing on what brought them to the child psychiatric inpatient unit and their relationships with each other. These are the families that I studied in depth as they participated in the parent-child group over the course of the children's hospitalization. Next, I will document how each of the three permanent leaders of the parent-child group over the course of my study viewed the group and their role as leaders. All of the narratives were developed from interviews and informal conversations with each participant.

THE BYRON FAMILY: WHY IS THIS HAPPENING?

Timmy

I'm seven years old. I came to the hospital because I told my father that I have a reflector in my head. I also gave my father a fat lip. My real parents are divorced. I used to live with my mother, but people in her family hurt me so I went to live with my grandparents (father's parents). Now I live with my father and Mary, my new mother.

Mike

I am Timmy's father. Timmy lived with my first wife and me for the first three years of his life. That wasn't good; I had a drinking problem. I'm a recovering alcoholic. I had Attention Deficit Disorder as a child and I was in treatment throughout most of my childhood, but treatment wasn't like it is now. I wish that doctors understood then what they understand now. Things would have been better for me.

My first wife and I divorced and Timmy lived with her until he was five. He said that he was getting hit by someone in my ex-wife's family and that two of his cousins sexually abused him. My parents took Timmy in for a year while I got my life together. Timmy has lived with me and my second wife, Mary, for about a year. Mary is planning on adopting Timmy. Things were great until about six months ago.

Timmy was out of control at home. All of his motor skills regressed. His ability to take care of himself was gone. We had to watch him every minute and we had to show him how to clean himself. We hospitalized him at a different hospital about five months ago. He was there almost a month, but nothing much changed. Just before he was admitted here, we found him smearing feces. He told a teacher that he wanted to kill himself. Timmy has a lot of his anger that is directed toward me. I get a lot of "I hate you. You're no good. You're not my father. You don't love me."

Before his first hospital admission, he would actually come at you. He hit, bit, scratched; he did whatever he could do to get you. If things don't go the way he wants, even when he's playing, he gets very upset. He'll break or smash things. He used to boast in school, "I beat up my dad!" Sometimes, he can sit in his room and be perfectly fine, but you can't predict that it's going to stay that way. You're always on the defensive.

You can't say no, you're not ever going to do anything with your child just because you're afraid that he is going to have a tantrum. That's just not right. You try and do things with him anyway, but you're always on the defensive. The first sign of anything going wrong, you react to it instantly and you either change the subject, get him out of there or you do whatever to try and cope with situation so your child doesn't have a full blown tantrum. It's not pleasurable to be with your kid. As things have gotten worse with Timmy, we've gotten more lenient. We stopped expecting more out of him. There were no expectations before he came to the hospital.

I can't connect with Timmy anymore. I can't reach him. The son that I have that's here today is not the son that I had six months ago. I don't know who that boy is in the other room. I don't know why this is happening.

THE NADLER FAMILY: OUR LIFE IS FALLING APART

Gary

I'm eight years old and I came to the hospital because I didn't listen to my mother. At home, I usually didn't do projects with my mother like I do here. We just played games sometimes, if my mother had the time. She didn't a lot because she always helps my brothers. I think that it's not fair for me. I have two brothers so she can't just play with me. I guess they have harder homework and I can do my homework by myself. I don't get time with her. When she's done helping them, she has to talk on the phone with her lawyer. She's getting a divorce. It makes me sad.

When my mother visits when there's no parent-child group, it makes me sad. She always talks to me about being in the hospital and doing bad at home. I have to stop fighting with my brothers.

Andrea

I'm not a bad mother, but maybe I've done things wrong. I've done all that I could and didn't expect the problems that I've had with my three sons. I took my kids to Mommy and Me classes; I went to parenting classes when I could find them. Doug is 14; he's been hospitalized for depression; he takes Prozac; he also has had lymphoma which is in remission. Billy, who is 10, has been hospitalized twice for depression and aggression; he needs to come back here. I'm trying to get him on the unit like Gary is.

Gary is 8, but he looks like he's 10 or 11. This is his fifth hospitalization in a year. I brought him here because he refused to go to school. He also is explosive, not as bad as Billy, but he's bad enough. Doctors also told me that he has depression.

I'm not a disciplinarian; I left that to my ex-husband. Now, I'm paying the price. I'm getting divorced, live in a one bedroom apartment with my three boys, lost my job and I'm on welfare. I've been a hostage in my home with Gary and Billy. They refuse to go to school, eat compulsively like my ex-husband's family, don't listen and fight really bad. Billy teases and beats on Gary without mercy; Gary has always been his target. I want to send them both to a residential school where they can get help. I can't keep bringing them back here. I need to get my life back together. My oldest son listens, goes to school and does his work. I want to get a job, go back to school and get off welfare.

THE SMITH FAMILY:
THEY BETTER FIND THE RIGHT MEDICATION

Joseph

I'm nine years old. I used to go to a special day school right here at this hospital. I live with my grandmother because my mother used to be mean to me. They put me in the hospital because I need a new medicine to help me pay attention. My old medicine was making my heart work funny.

When my grandma comes to visit, we play games like Candyland™. Today, we visited in the playroom. I played with a construction set; my grandma read me the instructions. I want to get on Level 3 so I can have a pass. I'm always on Level 1. Kids mess with me. I have to beat them up. I want to go home; I like being there. I like doing things with my grandma and other people in my family.

I liked it when my mother came to visit. She never comes to visit, just my grandma. She has to go a hospital like this to get help. She gets to have two roommates! That's no fair! Here, we have a room all alone or with only one other kid. When my mother came, it was better than with my grandmother. My grandma just says, "No, no, no, you can't do that!" She doesn't let me do anything. It's better with my mother! She brings me Puppet Master Comics. My grandma doesn't let me have them. She thinks they're too scary and violent! Same thing with movies! My mother lets me do everything!

Teresa

I'm Joseph's grandmother and I have custody of him. Joseph has lived with me on and off his entire life, but continuously since he was three. His mother, my daughter, Delia, is a drug addict. She treats Joseph different from her other kids. She has abused him badly.

I'm waiting for Joseph's behavior to improve. He's been hospitalized here three times. This is the second time this year. They have to find the right medication that will help him without causing heart problems. He just can't pay attention; he has attention deficit disorder and has been on many medications to help him. He also has to learn to follow rules. I keep telling him that grown-ups who don't follow laws go to jail. Joseph has always been explosive. He has had these fits of rage since he was about three. I used to hold him until he calmed down. Now he's getting too big for that. I took a course for parents on behavior management last spring. That was really helpful. One of the things that they taught me is that it's important to give a child a chance to get ready to come in the house when he's playing outside. Now, I tell Joseph that he has five more minutes before he has to come in; I used to just call him when I wanted him in the house. That didn't work as well.

It's hard for me when my daughter, Delia, visits Joseph because the visits are hard for Joseph. Maybe he remembers the violence and the abuse from the time that he lived with her. I think that he's afraid to get mad at her so he gets mad at me instead. He gets verbally abusive and sometimes he loses physical control with me when she's around. The next day, after she's gone, things go back to normal. Joseph has asked me if he could call me mommy. I told him no. I explained to him that everyone only gets one mother and he has one. He tells his brothers and sister that I'm "HIS grandmother" not theirs.

I like to spend time with Joseph alone when I visit. That way I can get him to concentrate and we can do things. I bring cards or the children's educational magazine, *Highlights*, to do when I come to visit.

THE THOMSON FAMILY: WE KNOW WE HAVE TO CHANGE, BUT WE DON'T WANT TO

Joshua

I'm nine years old. I was here in the hospital when I was six. I don't remember it much. After that I had to go to this residential school for a couple of years. It was okay, but I like living home better. I live with my mother and Bob. Bob has lived with my mother and me since I was four. My real father died from AIDS when I was three. That's what my mother told me. I don't remember. At home, I just like to watch videos and play videogames. I like to sit close to my mother and kiss her. I do that a lot with her. Sometimes, I wrestle with Bob; I like to pin him on the floor. That's fun!

Kathy

My son, Joshua, has been at home for the last year. I was so happy to have him home. He was in a residential school for children with emotional disorders for two years. He got better there; he was on the highest level when he left there. He was a star. I hospitalized Joshua here when he was just turning six because he was out of control. He was overactive and aggressive with me. He would hit me and pull my hair when he wanted attention. When he got angry, he destroyed things in the house; one time he pulled down all of the curtains in the house.

Since Joshua has been home this year, we just went along with everything and accepted what he did and that's it. Until it got too far out of hand. He doesn't do anything for himself when I ask him to, for instance to get dressed or to take a bath. He's always eating too, especially after school when he's with my mother. He was so little and skinny; now you can see the fat deposits on his neck. Even he doesn't like that! Joshua is fine unless you insist that he do something or if you don't give him what he wants, and then the whole confrontation ruins everything. He got very agitated with me which was a lot of the time because we had to do things. He hit me and broke things. We kept telling him that he'd have to go back to the hospital if he didn't stop hitting and didn't listen. I just said that this is too much. See these bruises all over my arms? These are from Joshua when we brought him to come here.

I feel that it's my fault though. I let him get away with things. I guess all parents do, but if you have a child with problems like Joshua, you can't treat him like a normal child. Joshua has always been hyperactive and he has been diagnosed with Pervasive Developmental Disorder. You have to run a strict home, like a school. I think that I didn't do it right. I feel guilt, but also anger. I'm a special education teacher and I know managing a child with a problem in school is easier. I want to see someone else manage Joshua at home and have him not do the things that he does. I'm angry that my home is going to have to be like a school. He'll have to earn everything he likes, television and videogames. That's the only way that he will do anything, but it feels sterile and not real.

To be strict with Joshua feels like less love, but it's going to have to be done. Joshua and I used to spend hours snuggling. I mean we would spend a whole half hour just hugging and throwing pillows. We can't do that anymore. He always says, "Can't I kiss you and talk to you at the same time?" He likes to kiss me a lot. I think that it's chivalrous, but all that kissing offends other people especially people here. I can tell by how cold people get to me on the unit when I get close to Joshua. I feel like they're telling me, "Your behavior has to change too!"

All I have for Joshua is hope. I'm not going to say that he's never going to change. That would be like saying I've given up on my child and myself. I think that he's going to grow out of this. Sometimes, I think that things won't get better. I see other mothers with their beautiful children and I compare them to me, but that's abusive to me.

doi:10.1300/J004v22n03_03

Chapter 4

One Parent-Child Activity Group:
A Framework and Snapshots

SUMMARY. The framework that the author developed for parent-child activity groups is described. This is followed by "snapshots" of a group session to enhance the readers' understanding of the framework. Excerpts of the author's logs from her participant observation of the parent-child activity group that she studied are organized sequentially to provide examples of each part of a parent-child activity group session. doi:10.1300/J004v22n03_04 *[Article copies available for a fee from The Haworth Document Delivery Service: 1-800-HAWORTH. E-mail address: <docdelivery@haworthpress.com> Website: <http://www.HaworthPress.com> © 2006 by The Haworth Press, Inc. All rights reserved.]*

KEYWORDS. Parent-child activity groups, group intervention, occupational therapy

THEORETICAL BASIS
OF A PARENT-CHILD ACTIVITY GROUP

Group theory suggests that therapeutic groups can have many benefits for participants including providing a powerful environment for

[Haworth co-indexing entry note]: "One Parent-Child Activity Group: A Framework and Snapshots." Olson, Laurette. Co-published simultaneously in *Occupational Therapy in Mental Health* (The Haworth Press, Inc.) Vol. 22, No. 3/4, 2006, pp. 33-47; and: *Activity Groups in Family-Centered Treatment: Psychiatric Occupational Therapy Approaches for Parents and Children* (Laurette Olson) The Haworth Press, Inc., 2006, pp. 33-47. Single or multiple copies of this article are available for a fee from The Haworth Document Delivery Service [1-800- HAWORTH, 9:00 a.m. - 5:00 p.m. (EST). E-mail address: docdelivery@haworthpress.com].

learning about others, for observing and imitating the behavior of others, and for facilitating members' sense of hope that a life situation can change by meeting others who have had similar problems and have overcome them (Yalom, 1995). Occupational therapy activity group theory combines these concepts from group theory with the central tenet of occupational therapy: that participating in purposeful activities in the here and now is critical to every person's mental health and is a powerful tool in fostering growth and adaptation in rehabilitation (Fidler & Fidler, 1978; Mosey, 1986). Engaging parents with their hospitalized children in everyday play or constructional activities might promote relaxed and productive interaction. This might, in turn, foster children's interest and ability to successfully participate in age appropriate activities, as well as provide the children with a means to gain their parents' positive attention. Parents might experience an increased sense of competence and control as they assist their children in successfully participating in activities. Parents and children might seek more opportunities to interact with each other in activities, after successful experiences within a structured group. The parallel participation of other families provides constructive examples and support beyond that provided by the group leaders. Old patterns of interacting may be examined and new ways to interact explored.

The literature on parent-child interaction suggests that the quality of interaction between parent and child is the result of the bi-directional influences of both parent and child (Bates, 1976; Bugental, Caporael & Shennum, 1980; Mash, 1984). This literature facilitated my thinking about the problem of interaction between parent and child, not as something that is the sole problem of a parent or a child. Many issues of both parent and child strongly affect how they will interact with each other.

Exploring the work of Murphy (1962) and that of other attachment theorists underscored the importance of engaging parents with their children in a way that both fostered pleasure and parents' sense of being competent in helping and soothing their children. In a longitudinal qualitative study of children from infancy through childhood, Murphy (1962) found that the most critical variables in how children developed coping skills were the quality of their mother's enjoyment of them and her active support and encouragement of them. Other studies found that children's confidence in their parents' availability was correlated with problem solving abilities (Matas, Arend, & Sroufe, 1978), social competence (Lieberman, 1977; Waters, Wittman, & Sroufe, 1979), and resourcefulness and perseverance in challenging tasks (Arend, Gore, & Sroufe, 1979).

My readings led me to develop guidelines for a parent-child group. What follows is how I conceptualized the parent-child group. I have continuously revised these guidelines based upon my readings and experience.

GUIDELINES FOR PARENT-CHILD ACTIVITY GROUP

There are four general purposes that I identified in setting up the group. It was designed to:

1. Ease tensions that occur around children's psychiatric hospitalization and lessen emotional estrangement between children and their parents by promoting pleasurable and reciprocal interactions between parents and children in structured play.
2. Increase children's interest and motivation for play by increasing their experience of their parents' interest and enjoyment of mutual play with them.
3. Increase the likelihood that parents and children will engage in mutual play activity in the future after they have positive experiences in mutual play with each other.
4. Increase parents' sense of competence in managing their children's behavior in mutual activity.

From reading related professional literature, I have chosen two guiding principles for the group. These were derived from professional literature that resonated with my experience in working with children who have been psychiatrically hospitalized. A key finding of Murphy's 1962 longitudinal study of children's play development was that the quality of parents' enjoyment of their children and their active support and encouragement of their children is critical to the children's development of coping skills. Preston (1990) found that parents of psychiatrically hospitalized children are likely to be much attuned to negative behavior and to be less sensitive to their children's positive behavior in the course of their interactions. These parents may not experience a sense of competence in managing their children's behavior. Neither these parents nor children may experience a sense of security, satisfaction, or pleasure in their interactions (Street & Treacher, 1986).

Many of these families may not have experienced relaxed and playful interactions for a long period of time prior to the children's hospitalization. Structured play that is supported and guided by therapists is potentially a medium through which a parent and child can experience or re-experience enjoyment of one another and impart mutual positive regard. Having multiple positive and successful play experiences and becoming aware of mutual activity interests may increase the likelihood that families will explore similar experiences outside of the parent-child activity group. It may also increase the parents' sense of competence in managing their children in mutual activity.

The parent-child activity group is a multifamily group where parents play with their own children parallel to other families under the guidance of two group leaders. Every week, families are introduced to specific, structured play activities in which all group members participate. They are provided with the opportunity to choose their own activities during the second half of the group.

The parent-child activity group is an open group in which new families may begin participating in the group when children are admitted to the unit. Families end their participation in the group when children are discharged from the unit.

All children who are hospitalized on the child inpatient unit are eligible to participate in the group. Children must be able to participate in activities in a group setting and their parents or other adult caregiver must attend the group with them.

The leaders' role is multifaceted. They structure the group environment by setting up the room prior to group, by choosing structured play activities and activities that families may choose for free play. During the group, key leader responsibilities are to assist families in adapting activities as necessary so that families can fully and pleasurably participate in activities, and to facilitate interaction between parents and children and among families participating in the group. The leaders also make suggestions to families when challenges arise in activities or interaction and model methods of limit setting, structuring children's activities, and monitoring children's level of stimulation when necessary. The leaders also cue parents and children so that they are able to make their wishes or concerns clear to one another. Prior to group sessions, leaders should talk with parents so that parental concerns about their participation or their children's participation in the group can be addressed. After group sessions, it is helpful for leaders to talk with parents about what occurred in the group.

The group session is divided into two parts. During the first part of the group, families participate in a structured play task that the leaders introduce. The leaders choose tasks that will likely be interesting to the participating children, but that also require some adult assistance to organize materials, plan the task, and/or carry out the task. Emphasis is on exploration of materials and elaboration of the initial ideas presented by the leaders rather than on correct implementation of a task or mastering technical skills. Examples of activities include paper mache, construction, and collages.

The group leaders begin each session by introducing new group members and then review and demonstrate possible ways to approach the structured play task. Examples of completed projects are also provided. Families are generally expected to participate in the structured play task for at least one half of the group before they can move on to free play. Exceptions are made when a child's psychiatric illness precludes engagement in a structured tabletop task for that length of time.

In the second part of the group, parents supervise or participate with their children in simple gross motor activities, board games, or play with tabletop toys that they choose with their children from among the materials available. The leaders help families to explore and find an activity that interests them.

Leaders inform families and children when there are 10 to 15 minutes remaining to the group session so that families can finish an activity. In the last five minutes of the group, parents and children put away the equipment and line up to return to the inpatient unit. Parents escort their children back to the unit and say goodbye to their children on the inpatient unit.

SNAPSHOTS OF A PARENT-CHILD ACTIVITY GROUP

To illustrate what a parent-child activity group session of the group just described might be like, the following snapshots of a parent-child group were developed from research data collected during my dissertation research study on a child inpatient unit at a major psychiatric hospital located outside a large northeastern city.

The hospital was built in the early 1900s when optimal psychiatric treatment was thought to best occur in a rural setting where patients could be immersed in activity. The hospital sits on 15 acres of manicured lawns. There are many small buildings around the campus. Ten of those buildings house inpatient and outpatient psychiatric units. In Smith Cottage, there is a children's inpatient unit that serves 17 children between the ages of 4 and 12 years. A few doors down from Smith Cottage, a stately gothic building, Winston Hall, has a large gym and a craft room on its main floor. Many children's activity groups occur in this building, including the parent-child activity group.

The group meets two times per week at a consistent time and in a consistent location. It typically meets on Monday and Wednesday evenings for one hour in Winston Hall. Families usually enter the group during the child's first or second week of hospitalization. Families are invited to attend both of the weekly groups. Some families do; for others, it is not possible due to other commitments.

Immediately prior to the parent-child activity group, parents gather by the locked door of the unit with their children who are hospitalized. Once all attendees are present, the group leaders escort them to Winston Hall. Once families arrive in the activities building, each family sits together in an area around a large square table. Supplies for an arts and crafts project are arranged in the middle of the table. A group leader introduces an arts and crafts project (using oven-bake clay to make animals, decorating picture frames) and demonstrates if necessary. Each family then begins to choose and collect the supplies that they need. As families work, the leaders observe the activity going on around the room, strike up conversation with group participants, and walk around the room and assist families as necessary. Projects typically take 30-40 minutes to complete.

After families finish their projects, they clean up the area that they worked in. Then a leader takes families into the gym; each family chooses a gross motor activity such as playing basketball or badminton. One leader remains in the group room with families that are still working on their projects. Leaders in the gym give families the equipment that they need and observe and monitor interactions among family members. One hour after the group begins, the leaders announce that it is time to put the equipment away for the evening and to go back to the unit. Parents walk their children back to the unit and say goodbye outside of the unit's door.

To help a reader visualize a parent-child group, I have organized excerpts from my logs sequentially from the time that parents and children gathered to go to group until parents said goodbye to their children. In some cases, there is more than one example about that time period of the group in order to share the ranges of interaction that I observed.

GETTING READY TO GO TO GROUP

It is Wednesday night about 5:55 p.m.; children are in their rooms for quiet time, a 30-minute period after meals for the children to calm down after the stimulating experience of a group meal. A nursing staff member sits in the darkened hall to make sure that all the children stay in their rooms. Maria, a parent-child group leader, sits typing reports into the computer in the nursing station. A nurse talks on the phone to a doctor while looking out the window of the nursing station onto the darkened and quiet hallway. At exactly 6 p.m., the unit's doorbell rings. No one gets up to answer the bell until the charge nurse says to the aide sitting in the hall that it is visiting time and she should let the parents in. Teresa, a custodial grandparent, nods to the aide and then walks into her grandson's room, shutting the bedroom door. A few minutes later, Beth, a recreational therapist and long-time group leader, bounces through the door on the other side of the unit and then into the nursing station. She asks the nurse if any families have arrived. The nurse reports that Joseph's grandmother is visiting him in his room. The doorbell rings again and it is Mike, Timmy's father, and Pat, Sam's mother. Sam left two weeks ago, but is back already! Beth scurries down the hall to intercept the parents before they walk into their children's rooms. She brightly announces that it's time for parent-child group. Then an aide calls to Timmy and Sam that their parents have come to visit and it is time for parent-child group.

Beth continues down to Joseph's room, knocks and opens the door and announces that it is time for group. Joseph and Teresa head towards the back door where the other families are waiting.

When Timmy sees Mike, his dad, he smiles, jumps onto his waist and gives him a big hug and kiss. Mike's tense facial expression softens and his smile reciprocally broadens; he seems equally happy to see Timmy. Sam walks up to his mother, asks her if she brought him snacks for his unit snack bag. She silently hands him a bag and he quickly looks inside. "Why did you bring this? I hate it!" In a monotone, Pat replies, "I'll take it back home." Sam changes his mind and says that he'll take the snacks anyway and hands the bag to an aide who says that he will put the snacks away for Sam. Sam turns to his mother and asks when he was leaving the hospital. Pat says that she doesn't know and that he has to work on his behavior before he could come home. Sam's sullen facial expression turns to a scowl and he slams his arms into a fold in front of his body. "She doesn't listen to me! Why do I have to be here? Everyone thinks that the problem is me! Well, it's her!" Pat shakes her head back and forth and quietly says to Beth who is standing next to her, "I come all this distance for this. This is what happens at home and I don't want to come if he acts like this. At home, he hit me when he got mad like this; I can't have him home if he acts like this."

Beth goes over to talk to Sam who is still glaring at his mother. Jane, the charge nurse, walks briskly down the hall and asks Beth about what was going on with Sam. They pull Sam away from the group and ask him if he thinks that he could talk to his mother nicely and attend group. Sam's face tightens, but then he nods yes. Beth walks through the group members gathered by the door, unlocks and opens the door. The group members follow her down the hall, out the cottage door, and down the path toward the activities building.

With his head down and his pace quick, Sam walks in front of his mother periodically turning around and saying things like, "It's always my fault when I get mad! It couldn't be that she does something bad! It's always me!" Pat keeps repeating that she can't take Sam home if he acts like this. She says that she doesn't want to take him home again and then have to bring him back the next day. Sam says, "I'm never going to come here again! If she tells me that we're going to a meeting at Green Hills, I'm not coming! She'll be trying to trick me!"

Timmy is not far behind Sam and his mother as they walk out the cottage door. He walks holding hands with his father. Timmy is looking out towards the parking lot. Mike is also scanning the parking lot ahead and he smiles when he sees his wife, Mary. "Look!" he exclaims to Timmy. When Timmy notices Mary, his smile becomes very broad. As Mary reaches the sidewalk, Timmy runs towards her and gives her a big hug. Mike waits for Mary and Timmy to catch up with him and then Timmy grabs both his and Mary's hands and the three of them walk toward the group building.

Joseph is walking a few paces behind Beth along with his grandmother, Teresa, and Christine, a group leader. Christine and his grandmother are talking about Joseph's last weekend pass. As they reach the path leading to the activities building, Joseph runs past Timmy and Sam, calling out, "I'll get there first!" He reaches the door and pulls on the door handle to open it, but the door is locked. "Hurry up!" he calls out to Beth.

INTRODUCING THE ARTS AND CRAFT PROJECT

At the beginning of each group, a leader introduces a different arts and crafts activity. Here are two examples of activities. Sometimes a leader directs families to plan a project around a family memory or everyday activity. Sometimes craft materials are presented in an open way, as in the second example.

Christine, a group leader, explains that tonight children would be making picture frames with their parents. She says that there were lots of puzzle pieces which they could use to make designs. After they make the frames, they should draw a picture of something that they like to do with their families. She asks if any of the children had made picture frames like this before. Jenny says that she made one in camp.

Beth introduces herself to the families stating that though she knows most of them, they might not know her. The children notice the Sculpey™ (soft oven-bake clay) in the middle of the table; Crystal asks if she could open it, Beth says yes. Beth says that she wants each family to take a quarter of a package of Sculpey™ and decide what they want to make together. The kids divide up the Sculpey™ by the time Beth finishes talking and are twisting it in their hands.

THE ARTS AND CRAFTS PROJECT

During project time, some parents and children have playful interactions around their project. For other families, project time is work for parents and children; children become quickly frustrated with the project and caregivers struggle with their children's frustration or limited task involvement. Some parents successfully engage their children; others do not. A few parents do not attempt to interact with their children and focus on their own craft.

> *Sculpey™*. Tom's dad asks Tom for a piece of Sculpey™ and uses the clay to shape a dog. He smiles as he tells Tom, "Check it out!" Tom smiles and takes the soft sculpture in his hand and exclaims, "Now watch this! Now, it is a dog lying down in the street and now it is a dog smashed by a car." Tom dramatically smashes the clay. His dad doesn't look upset, but says, "Come on and let's make something else." Tom says, "No, wait a minute, the dog needs tire tracks all over him." His dad shakes his head with a half smile, kneads the clay and gives Tom some. Tom says, "Let's make a rabbit," and then gets busy and focuses on shaping a rabbit. His dad has a little piece and makes a small animal. Tom looks up after a while, smiled at his father, then laughed and said "Dad, what's that? Are you making a rat?" The Dad looks back at him, smiles and says that he doesn't know. He says that he made a tail and then made an animal to go with the tail.

> *Banner*. Unlike some other nights, Joseph looks excited about making a banner with his grandmother, Teresa. He says that the Green Bay Packers are his favorite football team so he'd make a banner for that team. Teresa asks him how he wants to make the words on the banner. "Glitter, of course. You write the letters with the glue," he replies. Teresa obliges and after she writes each letter with glue, she stops, Joseph sprinkles on the glitter and then shakes off the excess glitter. Joseph works attentively, but periodically expresses frustration. As Joseph completes each letter, with a note of accusation in his voice toward his grandmother, he repeatedly states the letters aren't right. Each time, Teresa calmly shows him how they can easily fix the mistake. Sometimes he says that a letter doesn't look right no matter how Teresa reshapes it; Teresa calmly tells him to wait and see and they continue on to the next letter. Though at times, it looks like Joseph will pull out of the activity, each time he pulls away, he is pulled back in by his grandmother's coaxing, reassuring, and her calm fixing of mistakes. After the first word is completed, Teresa tells Joseph that it is his turn to write letters in glue. Gluing is a more challenging task for Joseph than sprinkling the glitter is. He hides his face in his arms after announcing mistakes in letter formation. His performance improves

with each letter and he seems reassured that his grandmother can resolve any mistake by the time they get to write the word, "Packers."

Suncatcher. Carlos sits to the left of his mom; his five-year-old sister sits on the mother's right. The mother's facial expression is hard to read, but she looks tense. Carlos' eyes are looking blankly into the distance out of the window. When his mother or a leader taps him and asks him to complete a part of the project, Carlos briefly focuses on the materials that his mother has placed in front of him. He cuts some strips of tissue paper for the sun catcher that they are making, but without continual adult coaxing, he drifts off the task at hand and resumes staring off into the distance. His sister stays involved in the activity. She works continuously alongside her mother. When she completes a part of the project, she talks with her mother about what she should do next or quietly watches her mother work.

Birthday Card. Jason, a nine-year-old child, quietly works on making a birthday card for his uncle. His mother sits next to him working on her own card for the uncle. "What are you making?" Jason asks. "What does it look like!" she retorts sarcastically. "It looks like one of those tattoos." "Well, it's not!" His mother seems emotionally cold and distant and primarily interested in doing her own card.

CONVERSATION

Sometimes, there is little or no conversation while families work on the project. Other times, there is lively conversation occurring between individual parent and child dyads, among families, between leaders and group members and among the children. Below are some examples of conversations that developed that were not related to the project.

Sisters. Jenny and her teenage sister, Kayleigh, are bantering back and forth with their aunt about their relationship. Their aunt says that Jenny looks up to Kayleigh, listens to her and likes to do what she does. On the other hand, they are always competing. Kayleigh says that Jenny never listens to her and that they just fight a lot. Christine, a leader, asks if she and Jenny ever get along; Kayleigh says yes, but she can't remember any times. While the conversation is going on, Shayna, an 11-year-old girl from another family, smiles and says that she and her sister do the same thing. Christine asks what she means; she says that her older sister says, "Hey, stop copying me!" Shayna's mother laughs and says that the conversation sounds all too familiar.

Children and a Parent. Sam says that if his mother was a good parent, he wouldn't be in a hospital. He says that the hospital is like a jail. He repeats this comment a few times. A few of the children giggle and the eyes of a few parents widen. Gary chuckles and calls out, "You're right! This is a jail!" Andrea, Gary's mother, shakes her head and says, "You don't know what a jail is! This hospital is a country club!"

Making friends. Wrestling comes up in the conversation between Joshua and his parents. He catches my eye and I smile at him. He brightens and says, "You know, I got to meet a lot of famous wrestlers!" His mother, Kathy, elaborates by adding that Joshua met the wrestlers at a stadium in a neighboring state. She takes out pictures of some of wrestlers from her pocketbook. Joshua then begins describing his favorite wrestler with animation. Joseph's eyes brighten and he asks Joshua if he could see the pictures. Joshua and Joseph then have a lively discussion about different wrestlers as they work on their projects with their families.

THE GYM

Children are expected to clean up their workspace and any supplies that they used before they can go into the gym or choose a table top game or toy. When children race into the gym without their families before cleanup, they are called back to the table by their parent or a leader. The leaders provide equipment, observe families play, and help set limits during gym time. Some families find ways to enjoy a gross motor activity together with or without a leader's assistance. For other families, the order and control of interaction that may have occurred during a structured craft project breaks down as they play in the gym.

Grandmother setting limits. When he finishes with his sand art picture, Joseph gets up and heads for the gym. Teresa strikes up a conversation with Beth, a leader, and doesn't notice that Joseph has gotten up until he is walking out the door. Beth calls him back to clean up with his grandmother. Joseph complies and quickly shoves a few pieces of cardboard into the middle of the table and gets up to leave. "That's not helping! If you can't clean up right, we'll just have to go back to the unit!" "Okay, Granny!" "You better believe me. I'll bring you back." Joseph then gets a sponge and cleans the sand off the table. He waits until Teresa is ready and then they walk into the gym together.

Negotiating play. Toward the end of the project, Tyrone asks his mother if he could play the piano that is in the foyer that separates the craft room and the gym. She says no, that they need to clean up and then wait for Beth to open the gym so that they can choose an activity to play in the gym. "Can't we play hockey like last week?" Tyrone playfully pleads. She gives a half-smile and says, "Of course." They shoot a plastic hockey puck back and forth for a few minutes; then Tyrone asks to play with a wiffle ball and bat. Betty nods. Betty pitches, and Tyrone is the hitter. Betty stands close to a wall and when Tyrone hits the ball, it bounces off the wall in his direction and he retrieves it. Betty is an older woman, probably in her sixties; she has a bad leg and walks with a cane. She doesn't look out of breath or stressed; she and Tyrone have found a way to play one of his favorite activities in spite of her physical limitations.

Anger exploding. Tonight is Joseph's second visit with his mother in about six months. Teresa, his grandmother, has managed to convince Delia to visit her son. Joseph, Teresa, and Delia are taking turns shooting basketballs. Joseph's sneaker becomes untied so he plops down on the basketball to tie it. Teresa grabs the basketball from beneath Joseph and resumes taking shots. Delia laughs as Joseph falls the short distance to the floor. Now sitting on the floor, Joseph screams, "She cheats! She's shooting while I'm tying my shoes! I hate her!" Teresa stops playing with the basketball and walks over the Joseph, tells him to stop yelling and to get up if he wanted to play. Ruth, a leader, begins walking toward the Smiths, but before she reaches them, a furious Joseph stomps out of the gym winging his arms in the air and cursing.

A parent and child face-off. Timmy and his dad are playing hockey. Earlier in the night, I had seen a boy who looked like he could be very active and might be disorganized if Mike didn't provide good structure, but he was well behaved. As I watch Timmy play hockey, he hits the puck in random directions; each time that the puck hits a wall, Timmy screams, "I got a goal!" His father tries to redirect him but has no success. When Mike moves in close to Timmy, Timmy hits Mike with the hockey stick on purpose. Mike grabs the puck to stop the game and tells Timmy not to do that again and that if they were playing with real sticks that Timmy would have really hurt him. Timmy stops for a minute, but then begins running around in circles; he hits his father again with his hockey stick, but this time with less force. Mike tries to stop Timmy, but Timmy keeps moving and swinging his stick in the air. Mike grabs Timmy. Timmy falls to the ground holding his knee and crying, "You hit me with your stick." Mike bends down and tries to console him. After Mike sits down on the floor next to Timmy, Timmy quickly gets up and starts to run around again. His tears are replaced by a laugh.

GOODBYES

For some children, goodbyes are warm closure to what appeared to be a night of positive interaction. For others, goodbyes feel heavy as children realize that it is time for their parents to go. At times, there are tears. Some children walk on the unit leaving their parents without any acknowledgment unless a leader directs them to go back and say good night.

A warm goodbye. Ruth tells Joseph and his grandmother that group is over. Joseph brings the ball and rackets back to the closet. His grandmother waits for him in the back; they walk to the front together. Both look a little tired; Joseph is sweaty. He snuggles up close to his grandmother who is smiling and put her arm around his shoulders. They walk back to the unit with grandma's arm resting on Joseph's shoulder.

Four goodbyes. It's time to go and Tyrone, Gary, and Timmy readily help with clean-up. Sam is resistive, but then helps. On the walk back to the unit, Tyrone walks close to his adoptive mother, Betty, and tries to be supportive as she walks. Once at the door to the unit, Tyrone warmly hugs his mother a few times and then asks her to call as soon as she got home. She says that if she can't get through tonight then she'll call tomorrow. He agrees and walks through the door onto the unit. Timmy hugs both his stepmom and dad and becomes tearful as he walks through the unit's door and away from his parents. Gary gives his mother a hug and then glumly clomps onto the unit. Sam looks down, mumbles goodbye after Beth asked him if he said goodbye to his mother and then walks quickly onto the unit.

REFERENCES

Arend, R., Gore, F. L., & Sroufe, L. A. (1979). Continuity of individual adaptation from infancy to kindergarten. A predictive study of ego resiliency and curiosity in preschoolers. *Child Development, 50,* 950-957.

Bates, J. E. (1976). Effects of children's nonverbal behavior upon adults. *Child Development, 47,* 1079-1088.

Bugental, D. B., Caporael, L., & Shennum, W. A. (1980). Experimentally produced child uncontrollability: Effects on the potency of adult communication patterns. *Child Development, 51,* 520-528.

Fidler, G. S., & Fidler, J. W. (1978). Doing and becoming: Purposeful action and self-actualization. *American Journal of Occupational Therapy, 32,* 305-310.

Greenfield, B. J., & Senecal, J. (1995). Recreational multifamily therapy for troubled children. *American Journal of Orthopsychiatry, 65,* 434-439.

Lieberman, A. F. (1977). Preschoolers' competence with a peer: Influence of attachment and social experience. *Child Development, 48,* 1277-1287.

Mash, E. J. (1984). Families with problem children [Children in families under stress]. *New Directions for Child Development, 24,* 65-82.

Matas, L., Arend, R., & Sroufe, L. A. (1978). Continuity of adaptation in the second year: The relationship of the quality of attachment and later competence. *Child Development, 49,* 547-556.

Mosey, A. C. (1986). *Psychosocial components of occupational therapy.* New York: Raven Press.

Murphy, L. (1962). *The widening world of childhood.* New York: Basic Books.

Murphy, L., & Moriarty, A. (1976). *Vulnerability, coping, and growth from infancy to adolescence.* New Haven, CT: Yale University Press.

Street, E., & Treacher, A. (1986). Developmental closure: A family systems approach to separation in residential care. *Maladjustment and Therapeutic Education, 4(2),* 42-47.

Waters, E., Wittman, J., & Sroufe, L. A. (1979). Attachment, positive affect and competence in the peer group: Two studies in construct validation. *Child Development, 50,* 821-829.

Yalom, I. D. (1995). *The Theory and Practice of Group Psychotherapy* (4th Ed.). NY: Basic Books.

doi:10.1300/J004v22n03_04

Chapter 5

A Qualitative Research Study
of One Parent-Child Activity Group

SUMMARY. The qualitative research methods used by the author to study one parent-child activity group are shared. This qualitative research study documented what the participants of a parent-child activity group on a child psychiatric inpatient unit reported about their experiences with each other and how these participants interacted with each other in the group over the course of eight months. The group was studied through persistent participant observation with formal and informal interviews of the participants throughout their participation in the group. The greatest benefit that some parents and children reported about their participation in the parent-child activity group was that the group opened a door to positive interaction between them that was not otherwise available during the children's psychiatric hospitalization. doi:10.1300/J004v22n03_05
[Article copies available for a fee from The Haworth Document Delivery Service: 1-800-HAWORTH. E-mail address: <docdelivery@haworthpress.com> Website: <http://www.HaworthPress.com> © 2006 by The Haworth Press, Inc. All rights reserved.]

KEYWORDS. Qualitative research, child psychiatric inpatient unit, parent-child activity group

---

[Haworth co-indexing entry note]: "A Qualitative Research Study of One Parent-Child Activity Group." Olson, Laurette. Co-published simultaneously in *Occupational Therapy in Mental Health* (The Haworth Press, Inc.) Vol. 22, No. 3/4, 2006, pp. 49-82; and: *Activity Groups in Family-Centered Treatment: Psychiatric Occupational Therapy Approaches for Parents and Children* (Laurette Olson) The Haworth Press, Inc., 2006, pp. 49-82. Single or multiple copies of this article are available for a fee from The Haworth Document Delivery Service [1-800- HAWORTH, 9:00 a.m. - 5:00 p.m. (EST). E-mail address: docdelivery@haworthpress.com].

My qualitative research study about parents, children and group leaders' experiences within a parent child activity group sought to answer the question: "What do the participants of a parent-child activity group report about their interactions with each other over the course of several months?" I used a qualitative research design to carry out this study (Bogdan & Biklen, 1992; Denzin & Lincoln, 1994; Ely et al., 1991; Ely, Vinz, Downing, & Anzul, 1997). Participants were members of the parent-child activity group on the child inpatient unit of a teaching hospital including children, parents, and three group leaders. I studied what naturally occurs in that group and interviewed participants about their interactions and experiences with each other. All names of people, places, and other identifiable data have been changed.

SETTING

This study took place on a child inpatient unit at what I will refer to here as Green Hills Hospital, a major psychiatric hospital located outside a large northeastern city. The hospital was built in the early 1900s when optimal psychiatric treatment was thought to best occur in a rural setting where patients could be immersed in activity. The hospital sits on 15 acres of manicured lawns. There are many small buildings around the campus. Ten of those buildings house inpatient and outpatient psychiatric units. In Smith Cottage, there is a children's inpatient unit that serves 17 children between the ages of 4 and 12 years. A few doors down from Smith Cottage, a stately gothic building, Winston Hall, has a large gym and a craft room on its main floor. Many children's activity groups occur in this building, including the parent-child activity group.

PARTICIPANTS

The children who participated in this study were between the ages of 5 and 11 years old and primarily males. They were hospitalized because they exhibited behaviors that endangered their own lives or the lives of others. Their psychiatric diagnoses included Depression, Oppositional Defiant Disorder (ODD), Conduct Disorder, Post-Traumatic Stress Disorder, Pervasive Developmental Disorder (PDD), Bipolar Disorder, Intermittent Explosive Disorder, and Attention Deficit/Hyperactivity Disorder (ADHD). Some of the children carried secondary diagnoses of learning and personality disorders. The primary caregivers who participated in this study were the biological or adoptive parents or relatives who had custody of the children who were hospitalized. I chose families whose children were hospitalized for at least one month. This permitted me to observe a family at least three times in the parent-child activity group, to complete at least two formal interviews with parents, and to have many informal conversations with them. The group leader participants were the regularly assigned leaders of this group.

I had the opportunity to observe many participants over the eight-month period during which I observed the parent child group at Green Hills Hospital. I observed and talked with 26 parent and child dyads, four group leaders, and two occupational therapy students. My observations and conversations with all of these participants contributed in some way to the description of the group setting and the wide focus of the experience of participants of this group. I observed 13 families in at least three groups. The other 13 families that I observed passed quickly through the unit and the group. Children arrived on the unit after a crisis, and they along with their parents were just getting acclimated to the unit during the first week of hospitalization. By the time they attended their first parent-child group during the child's second week of hospitalization, some had discharge plans for the coming week. There was often little time for establishing connections to the leaders or the other participants in the parent-child group. Many of these families only attended the group one time.

I observed families of different racial, ethnic, and socioeconomic backgrounds. Of the 26 families, one was Asian, 10 were African American, and 15 were Caucasian. The parents of one child were doctors, eight were middle socioeconomic status, and 17 had limited economic resources requiring public assistance and public medical insurance. The family constellations varied; there were two parent families, reconstituted families, single parents, adoptive parents, grandparents, grandaunts, and a granduncle. Ten of the children were reported to have had biological parents who abused drugs or alcohol and were physically abusive, neglectful, or failed to protect the children from sexual abuse. These children were presently being raised by other family members or by adoptive parents. When I talk in general about parents in this document, I am referring to all of the children's primary caregivers. I have done this to make my writing less cumbersome. When I refer to specific families, I specify each primary caregiver's relationship to children. See Table 1 for specific demographic and group-related information that may help readers understand the 13 children and caregivers whom I observed the most.

TABLE 1. Summary of Demographics and Number of Group Sessions Attended

Child's name	Age	Diagnosis	Caregiver attending group	Race	No. of groups observed
Joseph	9	ADHD; ODD	Grandmother and mother	African-American	10
Timmy	7	ADHD; Psychotic Disorder	Father and stepmother	Caucasian	8
Joshua	9	PDD, ODD	Mother and stepfather	Caucasian	4
Gary	8	Depression, Intermittent Explosive Disorder	Mother	Caucasian	5
Sam	11	Bipolar Disorder, Conduct Disorder	Mother	African American	3
Tom	11	Conduct Disorder, Depression	Father	Caucasian	3
Jason	10	Conduct Disorder	Mother	Caucasian	3
Jenny	9	ADHD, ODD	Grandaunt and uncle	Caucasian	4
Carlos	10	ADHD, Psychotic Disorder	Mother and stepfather	Hispanic	3
Tyrone	9	ODD, Depression	Adoptive mother	African American	4
Rasheem	10	Conduct Disorder	Grandaunt (adoptive mother)	African American	4
James	10	Conduct Disorder, Depression	Adoptive father	African American	3
Brian	10	ADHD, Depression	Mother and father	Caucasian	3

Note: ADHD = Attention Deficit Disorder, ODD = Oppositional Defiant Disorder, PDD = Pervasive Developmental Disorder

From the leaders, I learned about staff's perceptions about each family's background. From parents in these families, I learned about how the parents understood their children, their interactions with their children, and the parent-child group. Children shared their views with me about participating in parent-child group with their primary caregivers. I talked with some parents as they sat in the hall outside of the unit waiting for visiting hours to begin. I most frequently talked to three parents and one custodial grandparent and their children. I observed them at least four times in parent-child group, interviewed the parents and the grandparent two times formally and talked with them regularly before and after groups. I also interviewed each of the children one time and talked to them informally in the dayroom after groups. My experience was that formal interviews were difficult for the children. Though I completed three formal child interviews, I gathered more information about the views of the children from casual conversations that I had with them during their free time on the unit.

GENERAL PROCEDURES

This qualitative study involved participant observation, informal interviews, and audiotaped formal interviews of parent, child, and group leader participants. After the study was approved by the University Committee on Activities Involving Human Subjects of the Office of Sponsored Programs at New York University and the Institutional Review Board at the Hospital where the study occurred, I sought and received informed consent from the group leaders. I then began participant observation of the parent-child activity group weekly and interviewed the leaders about their perceptions of the group. After observing four group sessions, I began to approach parents to seek their interest in participating in interviews for this study.

Once one or two parents and children agreed to participate in the interviews with me, I completed the interview process with those parents and children and my concurrent analysis of the data that I collected from those interviews before I began interviewing additional parents and children. This took between three and four weeks. I interviewed parents and children while I continued my participant observations. I stopped my participant observation along with my interviewing of participants when my data began to repeat itself. This occurred in 8 months.

RECRUITMENT

When I first met with the two group leaders who were initially the only leaders of the group, I explained to them that I was requesting their permission to observe their group weekly for a period of three to six months and to interview them at least three times over the course of the study. At that time, I also gave the group leaders a cover letter describing this study and requested their permission to audiotape interviews with them relative to their experiences as leaders of parent-child activity groups. I guaranteed that their discussions with me were confidential and that I would not identify them by name, place of employment, or geographic location in my dissertation or in any publications that may develop as a result of this study.

After the group leaders gave their informed consent for my participant observation, I began to observe the parent-child activity group. Before each group meeting began, a group leader asked the participants
whether they consented to my observing the group that evening. If any
participants did not consent to my observing the group on a particular
night, I would not have observed the group that evening. Participants
gave consent for my observing the group during each week of my participant observation.

Attending four groups before approaching parent group members
about participating in interviews allowed me to orient myself to the
group and its members and become a "familiar stranger" (Ely et al.,
1991). I sat at the group table with the families and group leaders and
quietly observed. During gym time, I sat on a bench along the gym wall
close enough to observe the group's participants. I worked not to intrude on family activity or conversation. I learned about the structure of
the group at the time, how activities were used, and how group members
interacted with each other. My participant observation also gave me the
opportunity to consider questions that I wanted to ask participants during interviews.

I approached parents individually after they had attended their first
parent-child activity group and asked if I could speak to them for about
five minutes about a research study related to the parent-child activity
group. I re-introduced myself as a doctoral student doing a research
study about the parent-child group for her doctoral dissertation and in-
quired about the parent's interest in learning about this study. This occurred before or after a parent-child group. Parents and children had
already met me at an earlier time since I was a participant observer in the
parent-child activity group. If parents were interested in learning more
about the study, I arranged a meeting with them at a mutually convenient time so that I could explain the purpose and methods of the study
to them. I stated that I was working on a study about what parents, children, and group leaders report about their interactions with each other
during the parent-child activity group. I explained that I was observing
the group for a few months, and that during that time, I also would like
to talk with parents and children about their experiences in the group so
that I could understand the group from different points of view. I also
gave parents a cover letter that summarized my research.

I also explained to parents that it was their right to refuse to participate without any effect on their experiences at the hospital where this
study took place and their right to terminate participation at any time.
The confidentiality of all information shared was also described. Par-

ents who were interested in participating were given a copy of the informed consent form. If they decided to participate, they verbally
informed me of their decision on their next visit to parent-child group
and then I asked them to sign an informed consent form in the presence
of a witness who was a unit staff member not involved in the parent-child group. The witness and I also signed the informed consent. I
then filed the signed informed consent in a locked file cabinet. Parents
were told that now their children would be asked if they wished to participate in the study.

I talked with the hospitalized children of parents who agreed to participate and gave permission for their children to participate. The children's assent to participate was sought. Similarly, I re-introduced
myself to children individually at a free time on the inpatient unit and
ask if they were willing to talk to me about the study. If children agreed,
I explained the study to them by telling them that I was studying what
parents, children, and group leaders think about the parent-child activity
group. I explained that I was observing the group for a few months and
would talk to them about their experiences in the group. I confirmed
with children that they had the right to refuse to participate without any
effect on experiences at the hospital. They were also told that they had
the right to terminate participation at any time and that confidentiality of
all information shared was assured.

In families where both parents attend the group together, I gained
permission from both parents. I interviewed a biological father and
stepmother, a biological mother and two stepfathers, several single
mothers, and a custodial grandmother.

INTERVIEWS

At the initiation of my study, I interviewed the two therapists who
were the sole group leaders at that time; I formally interviewed them
two additional times in order to learn more about their perspectives of
the parent-child group, their role within the group, their view of the families with whom they were working, to ask for clarification about data
that they had already offered me, and to share my understanding of what
they shared with me so that they had the opportunity to correct any mis-
understanding or to verify my interpretations. One leader, Christine,
met with me three times during her two months as a leader; her family
relocated to another geographic area of the United States and she left the
hospital. I interviewed Beth three times formally over the eight months

of my study and informally talked with her after numerous groups. Ruth began to lead the parent-child group six months into my study. I interviewed her formally in the eighth month of my study and informally from the beginning of her leadership until the end of my study.

I used a list of interview questions that I developed as a means to promote and guide interviews, but once the interview was initiated, I followed the directions of the data that the leaders intended to share with me on a particular day. During my first interview with the leaders, I asked about their tenure as group leader, general impressions about the group, their role within the group, and any experiences interacting with parents and children within the group that stood out in their memory. In my subsequent interviews, I asked questions specifically about their experiences within the group since our last interview, including how they perceived their interactions with individual families. Based upon their responses to my initial questions during an interview, I asked probing questions about the topic or topics that seemed most relevant to them on a particular evening so that they described their experiences in depth to me.

I initiated my first formal interview with the group leaders after observing the parent-child group one time. One was a recreational therapist and the other was one of the social workers for the child inpatient unit. I interviewed them separately because this was most convenient for them. They played distinct roles within the parent-child group and on the unit. The recreational therapist, Beth, led the group for five years. She was responsible for maintaining the structure and organizing the group on a weekly basis. The social worker, Christine, had joined the group six months prior to my study; she was primarily hired to co-lead the group and to be responsible for talking with the children's primary therapists and nurses so that she and Beth could also focus on concerns with parent-child interactions that these other clinicians noted.

I chose families to interview in depth based upon their willingness to participate in formal interviews. I formally interviewed four parents at least twice, and I informally talked with them after each group that they attended which I also observed. The number of times that I interviewed each parent participant depended upon their availability, the information that they offered me, and any additional questions that grew out of my data analysis. One parent chose not to have her interviews with me audiotaped. The child participants tolerated only short interview periods; their interviews ranged from 10 to 30 minutes in length.

I interviewed participants in ways and in places that they appeared most comfortable. I met with the recreational therapists and social worker in an office on Smith Cottage. I met with children in the unit day room, in their rooms during a quiet period after dinner, or in a small playroom on the unit. I met with parents in Winston Hall after parent-child groups, in a quiet room on Smith Cottage, or in a quiet area in a courtyard on the hospital grounds. Some group participants did not wish or were unable to participate in lengthier, audiotaped interviews because of time constraints, but were willing to talk to me during my participant observation. What they shared with me enhanced my understanding of what I observed in the group by supporting or challenging my perceptions of what I observed or heard. Other parents seemed more open to me when I met with them informally as they sat with other parents waiting to visit their children. The latter provided me with a different perspective as participants shared their thoughts among themselves.

There were times when participants were open to talking with me while we were waiting for all group members to gather on the unit before going to the group room, during group transitions from structured activity to free play, during a short break from a gross motor play, or when we walked back to the unit after the group. Much of the data collected during participant observation are based upon informal interviewing (Fontana & Frey, 1994). These interactions helped me establish rapport with participants, and good rapport naturally leads to more informed research (Fontana & Frey, 1994). In addition, participants had spontaneous thoughts about interactions that just occurred which they might not have remembered when a scheduled interview occurred a week later or that they might have viewed differently after time passed. Comparing participants' perceptions at different points in time helped me to better understand the complexities of their perspectives.

The purpose of doing an in-depth interview "is to learn to see the world from the eyes of the person being interviewed" (Ely et al., 1991, p. 58). I learned how participants see the other members of the group and how they experienced participating in the group itself. I used interview methods typically employed by qualitative researchers with open-ended questions to lead participants to share important information that would not be discussed if the questions were close-ended. During my first interviews with parents, I asked them to tell me about their experiences in the parent-child activity group. Based upon what seemed most relevant to them on the particular evening, I asked probing questions to learn more about their specific perceptions and experiences related to the structured and free play part of the parent-child activity group and how it compared to their experiences with their children in activity at home and at other visiting times. In subsequent interviews, I asked about their experiences in parent-child activity group since their last conversation with me. I sought specific descriptions of their interactions with their children, the group leaders, and other families during the group, as well as descriptions of their interactions with their children at other times during the hospitalization.

The interviewees were full partners in my research process (Ely et al., 1991). I had a clear direction of where I desired to go throughout the course of an interview, but I did not rigidly control the interview content. My initial interview questions were focused on the few issues described above. In this way, I did not overly focus my interviews on many details and my participants had room to tell their story (Bogdan & Biklen, 1992; Wolcott, 1995). As an interviewer, I worked to be conscious of the power of active listening to facilitate a speaker's effectiveness (Wolcott, 1995). I asked clear questions to initiate discussion and asked follow-up questions to prompt the interviewees to talk more about particular topics that they brought up that I was interested in learning more about (Bogdan & Biklen, 1992). I worked hard to speak judiciously and focused my energies on listening. To be fully present with my study's participants, I did not write notes during interviews or participant observations. I audiotaped formal interviews when participants permitted. Upon returning to my home immediately following an interview or observation, I wrote extensive field logs about my experiences.

All audiotaped interviews were transcribed. A paid professional did transcriptions during the week following an interview. In order to insure the accuracy of these transcriptions, I reviewed each transcript word for word while listening to the audiotape. After I made necessary corrections to a transcript and inserted observations, I began coding it and comparing that data with the data and codes from my completed field logs, interviews, and analytic memos.

PARTICIPANT OBSERVATION

Participant observation was an important method of data collection for this study. It requires "the interweaving of looking and listening, watching and asking" (Lofland & Lofland, 1984). I attempted to make the familiar unfamiliar, and the unfamiliar familiar (Ely et al., 1991). This means that I did not assume that I fully understood what was occurring based upon my prior experiences of leading parent-child groups. It also means that I continuously observed and reflected on what were unfamiliar behaviors or perceptions to me in order for them to become familiar enough so that I could use those observations to facilitate my learning about the meaning of what occurred to the participants. Observation of participants' nonverbal behavior in the group provided me with data that at times corresponded and at other times, contradicted what I heard or saw. By reflecting on my participant observations, I enriched my understanding of the participants and developed hunches to explore in interviews with them.

I began this study with a wide focus (Lincoln & Guba, 1985) by observing all the participants in the group. This gave me the opportunity to learn about the range of experiences of different participants in the group, to orient myself to the particular group, and to sharpen my research focus. Participant observation enriched what I learned interviewing participants. I was able to reflect upon what I observed in contrast to what they reported. My observations provoked questions that I pursued when I was able to talk with participants after groups. My observations became more focused and selective over time as I searched for data that were related to questions raised by my prior observations and participant interviews (Spradley, 1980).

Group attendance varied during the eight months of this study. At times there was one family, sometimes three or four families, and a few times five or six families attended the group. I observed five groups in which only one family attended. I did not attend some groups toward the end of my study when there was only one family because there were professional students participating or observing the group in addition to one or two leaders. This number of observers seemed overwhelming to families even without my participation. This occurred primarily in the last two months of my study. Groups with three or more families occurred in the first three months of my study and in the sixth month. There were times when no families showed up to visit their children and therefore the parent-child group was canceled. This occurred six times over the course of my participant observation from the second month to the eighth month.

DATA MANAGEMENT

Field logs are the "repository" of all data that are collected during a qualitative study (Ely et al., 1991). All of my interviews, notes about participant observations, and analytic memos comprise my field logs.

During the entire study, I wrote about my ongoing group observations; I wrote about what I observed and about my own participation. Audiotaped interviews were transcribed and became a part of my ongoing field log. Analytic memos were written about my own feelings and insights about my field and interview experiences, about re-entering a system and a group where I had previously worked for ten years, and about how my role as a participant observer evolved.

Once I began interviewing participants, I wrote analytic memos about my reactions to the experience and my thoughts about what was said immediately following the interview. This was an important step in establishing my trustworthiness and credibility since it allowed me to carefully examine my own biases and separate them as much as possible from my field data. Regular writing of analytic memos served as a tracking system of how my thinking about this study evolved. Lincoln and Guba (1985) describe analytic memos as being the audit trail. They are the means of tracing the evolving conceptual thinking of the researcher and to assist the researcher in seeing gaps in the researcher's thinking. My logs served as a chronological record of what I observed and heard, as well as what I thought and read related to my study. My early hunches and conceptualizations about what my data might mean to me were recorded in analytic memos.

I wrote my field logs on a word processor. I used wide margins so that I could write notes to myself in the margins. Pages were consecutively numbered and lines on each page were also numbered in order to support data retrieval.

DATA ANALYSIS

I used a recursive method to analyze my data; I compared new data with data previously collected. I looked for similarities in the tentative categories of my old data or whether new data challenged the old or brought up new issues. By comparing old data with new data, the potential meaning of old data became clearer and raised new questions about the similarities and differences between the data. The old data provided a foundation for viewing the new data.

Field logs contain two kinds of material, descriptive and reflective (Bogdan & Biklen, 1992). I provided ongoing descriptions of my participant observations, as well as of my experiences interviewing participants. It was important that they were detailed and provided clear pictures of my perceptions of what I saw and heard. The substance of my data analysis began within these logs (Ely et al., 1991). I also included observer comments (OC) bracketed off within my field logs so that I could reflect upon my feelings and biases about what I observed. It was important that I separated my opinions from what I actually saw or heard. This allowed me to go back to my logs and explore whether any of my own feelings, opinions, or biases were getting in the way of my seeing and hearing the participants and being fair in my analyses. I did this many times throughout my analyses of my data and wrote analytic memos about my feelings and opinions versus the data.

Coding. "Analysis involves working with data, organizing them, breaking them into manageable units, synthesizing them, searching for patterns, discovering what is important and what is to be learned and deciding what you will tell others " (Bogdan & Biklen, 1992, p. 153). Coding is the first step in this process. It involves taking apart an observation or a sentence or paragraph from an interview and giving it a name. I developed tentative codes to begin my analysis after my initial group observations. As my analysis progressed, I refined my coding system and developed new codes to best name sections of data.

Codes are compared with other codes to look for relationships and differences among them. Questions are also asked about the codes after which they are lifted to a higher level of abstraction, categories (Strauss & Corbin, 1990). Categories not only help organize data, but help the researcher discover themes within and across categories.

Analytic memos provide the researcher with "room for integration and speculation" (Ely et al., 1997). They are written throughout the research process so that the researcher reflects on the study's focus, possible biases, initial insights about how pieces of data might fit together, and what the essence of the participants' perceptions might be.

Analytic memos are a critical part of recursive analysis. Recursive analysis refers to the intertwining of data collection and analysis. The researcher reflects on the data that have been collected while collecting more data. The analysis of data informs future data collection (Ely et al., 1991). At times, I only realized through the process of writing an analytic memo that in order to clarify my developing interpretations, I needed to focus on observing particular interactions among participants in subsequent participant observations. I developed themes about my data that I tested during subsequent observations and interviews. Participant comments or behaviors provoked new questions that I felt were important to pursue.

Through my analytic memos, I also explored ethical dilemmas that arose due to the nature of my study. I had differences of opinion with the group leaders on how to best facilitate interaction within and among families. I wrote about my thoughts so that I became clear on what the differences were. I observed parental and leadership behavior that appeared neglectful to me. I also wrote about my feelings and about the times that I stepped out of my researcher's role. I found myself feeling more positive and compassionate toward some participants than others. I reflected on these feelings as they arose so that I was able to develop as deep an understanding as possible of the participants.

Themes are statements that focus the reader on the essence of the data and the relationships among categories (Ely et al., 1997). They may express a central issue or concern about a particular participant's experience or may address key issues that may be common among several participants' experiences. I became aware of preliminary themes after I coded and categorized data into bins. I searched for themes that expressed the essence of the categories that I developed and that expressed the connections between specific categories. These themes were challenged by new data and by my continual analysis of all of my data. To become more in touch with the perspectives of particular participants as well as my own perspectives, I wrote narratives about incidences that I observed, vignettes about particular participants, and poems taken directly from my data. These writings facilitated my developing themes about the participants whom I studied in depth. In this way, I discovered the essence of what was important about the parent-child group to different participants of a parent-child activity group.

Metathemes are overarching themes that are reflective of all of the data collected within a study (Ely et al., 1991). In this chapter as well as in the next, I introduce metathemes that I developed to describe what I experienced as the essence of the parent-child group for its parent and child participants. These metathemes evolved through my analysis of the similarities and differences in the viewpoints of parents, children and group leaders over the course of their participation in the group during the time period of my study. I have used the metaphor of a door opening or being blocked to describe what I observed about the interaction of parents and children during their participation in the parent-child activity group. In Chapter 7, I describe a metatheme that lifts my analysis beyond parent-child activity group. This metatheme emerged during my final analysis and interpretation of the data as I considered how the culture of the parent-child activity group as a therapeutic activity group offered at an inpatient psychiatric hospital impacted the way in which parents and children participated in the parent-child activity group.

TRUSTWORTHINESS AND CREDIBILITY

Trustworthiness and credibility in qualitative research refer to the researcher striving to capture the experience of the participants as accurately as possible in the study's findings. Because the qualitative researcher is the research instrument, it was important that I examine myself in the research process to establish trustworthiness and credibility in my research.

Prolonged engagement and persistent observation mean that I sufficiently engaged in the field of my study and conscientiously observed the events and interactions that occurred. I observed the parent-child activity group in process over the course of eight months and interviewed each participant at least twice. I observed the participants in the group and talked with them informally before group, after group, or when I met them on the unit. I knew that I had observed sufficiently when my data and themes became repetitive, as opposed to becoming more elaborate and changing (Lincoln & Guba, 1985). When my data collection ended, I maintained a relationship with the parent-child activity group while I worked on my data analysis and interpretation. Going back to the group a few times after I finished my data collection gave me confidence in my data analysis, provided me with the opportunity to ask the leaders new questions that developed as I wrote, and raised new questions and led to deeper analyses when I observed interactions that were consistent or contrasted with what I was writing.

Support Group. I participated in a support group with four other doctoral candidates who were also using qualitative methods in their doctoral research. I had the opportunity to share my raw data and my reflections and interpretations of that data throughout my study. I charged my support group with the job of carefully reading my researcher's stance and examining my data and my analysis for evidence of blind spots. I shared portions of my field logs, interview transcripts, and analytic memos with these peers. They shared their thoughts with me on the direction that I took in my ongoing data analysis. They challenged my approach to the data collection and help me to see past personal blind spots. By questioning me about my research process and my feelings about what I heard and observed, I was helped to be as open as possible to learning from the participants. As I engaged in preliminary analysis of my data, my peers examined the merit and the consistency of my thinking and challenged my interpretations, and shared their alternate interpretations of my data. My peers also led me to explore how I presented my data. They made me more aware of the reader over my shoulder.

Participant Checking. I also presented some of my findings to the persons that I observed to check for the accuracy of those findings. I had a minimum of two interviews with each participant. During the second interview, I asked participants for clarification of some thoughts that they shared with me and I reviewed with them how I understood what they told me in their first interview. I listened carefully to their responses so that I could enhance my understanding and to correct any inaccuracies in my developing presentation of their viewpoint. I shared the tentative themes that I developed based upon my particular experiences observing them in the group and through my conversations with them. In this way, I checked if my themes resonated with my participants or whether I needed to reconsider how I interpreted the data.

Peer Review. A former employee of Green Hills who led the parent-child group for 10 years prior to my study read drafts of my work and provided specific feedback to me about what resonated for her in my written work about the parent-child group. Her critical comments facilitated my deeper thinking about therapists' interactions with parents and children.

Negative Case Analysis. As I analyzed the data and develop themes, I looked for incidents or cases that challenged the accuracy of those themes. This is an important technique because it guides the researcher to critically examine findings and reanalyze them in light of negative cases that occur. In this way, the final themes that I present are as true to the data collected as possible.

FINDINGS OF STUDY

Parents and children reported that participating in the parent-child activity group provided them with an opportunity to interact in a positive way through activity that was not otherwise available during their child's psychiatric hospitalization. They also reported that their interactions were different from the ways that they had been interacting with each other prior to the hospitalization. The greatest benefit for the parents and children was that it had the potential to open a door to positive interaction between parents and children who struggled with each other prior to the child's hospitalization.

A Door Is Opening

Having the structure of a group to encourage interaction in play activities seemed to help some parents and children spend time together. The organization of the group and the presence of the leaders and other families enabled some parents and children to approach each other differently. One mother said, "Before he came here, I yelled at him a lot. He don't listen. We didn't spend a lot of time doing things together. He watched a lot of videos. It's nice to sit down and do things with him." For others, some experiences in the parent-child activity group seemed to give parents new insight into their relationship with their children.

Though the leaders state that the parent-child group provides an opportunity to see how family members really interact with each other, parents and children reported that their interactions with each other are different in the group than they are at other times. When a family walks through the door of the group, they enter an environment where an activity is set up for them, and where support for benign or positive interaction in activity is available. Many of the people who are also present in the group are new to them or are people that they just met in passing. Family members are expected to engage in joint activity in the presence of leaders and other families and generally follow as they see the other families around them engaged in joint activity. Parents and children reported that their interactions in such an environment were different from their interactions in private, familiar settings. Mr. Mendez, the stepfather of one nine-year-old boy said,

> There's no hostility, no yelling or screaming. Everything is working nice and smooth. I wish things like this could work in real life, but it just doesn't happen like this. Carlos knows that there's supervision here. I guess kids become a little more apprehensive about really showing their true colors as opposed to just being home with mom and dad.

With different interactions in a different and somewhat public environment, there is the opportunity for parents and children to make new connections with each other. Some parents found that they began to relax and have fun with their children whom they felt held them hostage at home. At the beginning of Timmy's hospitalization, his father Mike stated:

It's hard. It's exhausting to do an activity with him. It's not pleasurable because you're focusing all of your attention and energy on watching his behavior and not on playing the game. You're putting all that extra effort out on watching him so that he doesn't have a tantrum, or get upset or angry. You really have to watch what you do, how you say things and how you react towards him. You let your guard down for a minute and as soon as you do, he's in a tantrum or acting up. So you stop letting your guard down. You're always jumping up and saying, "No! Don't do that!" Sometimes, it's not his fault, but you're always hovering over him because you just don't know what he'll do.

Over the course of a month, Mike said, "Parent-child group is fun. It's very relaxing to sit here and do projects with Timmy. I didn't feel like this a few weeks ago. He's doing well in this hospital."

It Gives Us a Chance to Interact

Children reported happily anticipating their first parent-child group. They were able to leave the unit and got to do something fun with their families while the children who don't have visitors take showers. Children's comments focused on being with their families and doing activities that they enjoyed.

Joseph said: I like going to parent-child group. You get to do things that you don't get to do on the unit like doing projects and playing in the gym. Sometimes, you get to do that stuff with kids on the unit, but it's better in parent-child group because you get to do it with your family.

Joshua's comments echo Joseph's words: "I like coming to parent-child group. Playing in the gym is fun; I like doing the projects. I get to make what I want with my mother. It's better than doing things on the unit."

Timmy's comment brought up an added potential benefit of working with parents. Parents often help children make the projects to the child's specifications.

Parent-child group is good. You get to do things with your parents. You could play. I made a suncatcher with my parents. I did the work. They helped a little bit. I told my parents how I wanted to make it and we made it that way.

For some children, like Gary, the parent-child group is their primary contact with their parents while they are hospitalized. He commented:

> Going to parent-child group is good. You get to do activities and stuff. That's the only time that my mother visits. I made a sun-catcher and I painted a car. My mom is going to come tonight and we are going to finish painting a car.

Initially, some of the parents expressed uneasiness about going to the parent-child group. They said that they felt that hospital staff would watch them and would evaluate how they worked with their children. They stated that they just wanted to visit with their hospitalized children and not be bothered with staff and having to participate in a group. Some didn't expect that participating in an activity group with their children could be a pleasurable experience since they expected that their children would be as difficult to engage as they were at home. Mary, Timmy's stepmother, said:

> At first, I felt like there were people watching over us. What were they looking for? What were they trying to see? I wished that girl who was an occupational therapy student would just sit down and ask me about my day. She stood there with her arms folded and stared down at everyone. It made me feel like I was under a micro-scope. Well, maybe not to that extreme, but it makes you feel un-comfortable, at least when you first start the group.

Once having attended the group, some parents describe it as a welcome relief to looking at the four walls of their children's room and as a chance to do something productive. Timmy's father, Mike, commented:

> It took us a few times to get used to the group. It was harder for me to go to the group than to visit on the unit with Timmy. He got rest-less working on a project for so long and wanted things his way. He needed a lot of structure, reinforcement and direction. When he didn't have it, like in the gym, it was a free for all. Timmy has got-ten better while he's been here. Timmy and I really like par-ent-child group now. It's a group where you can do things and have fun with your child. It's different.

Besides experiencing her child as easier to manage, Kathy spoke about using activity as a way to interact with her child. At home, Kathy described being very involved with Joshua in everyday physical care even though Joshua is nine. She made sure that he was properly washed which she described as meaning that she physically cleaned him in the bath. She regularly washed and combed his hair as well. She said that Joshua should manage his personal care independently, but he wasn't doing it as well as she thought it should be done, so she did it. In free time at home, Kathy described Joshua as very involved in computer games or watching videos. He became very upset, yelled at her, and at times threw objects around the room if she interrupted his activities. She found it easier to let him participate in his favorite activities unless she needed to take him on an errand or if it was mealtime. She spent time with Joshua hugging and kissing him like "her baby." Though she enjoyed this, she has decided that this has to change if she is going to be able to manage him at home and get him to act like a nine-year-old boy. She commented:

> Arts and crafts are a good way to get you and your child talking in general. The last time, Joshua was really interacting with Joseph. He doesn't do that. He's never had a real friend. He was talking to Joseph like a friend. Maybe, they'll play together on the unit.

We Interact Differently

Attending the group was a different experience for parents and children. Parents' and children's expected behaviors are implicitly and explicitly different in the group than when they interact on the unit or in sessions with therapists or social workers. In the parent-child group, they are not asked to talk about their problems, but to do something positive together like complete an arts and crafts project or play a game together. They are required to stay together and to work as a family; children are not permitted to play with other children or leave their parents. Parents may talk intermittently among themselves, but they are asked to remain engaged with their children in an activity. With leaders and other families present, family members may be more subdued and act in ways that seem socially acceptable in a group environment. This may be different from their usual interactional patterns with each other.

Group members typically acquiesce to the group mores. Some report that they have not been involved in leisure activities like this with each other before. With surprise, one mother stated, "I have to take out all of my craft supplies when I'm home with my kids. It's nice to see how focused and how well they get along with each other when they are engaged in their own project." The father of a child who was diagnosed with Oppositional Defiant Disorder said that the group "is a different experience because you are forced to be considerate of one another and not just bark at each other."

One mother noted, "Kids are on their best behavior." She said this with a smile, as if this environment made it possible for her to enjoy her child for now even if she didn't experience the child's behavior as typical.

Gary's mother, Andrea, stated:

> It's the only time that I'll visit my son. He never pays attention to me on the unit. He says that he wants to visit on the unit, but then he gets involved with the other kids. Parent-child group gives me quality time with Gary. We get to do something together, even if he rushes through the project to get to the gym.

> We haven't done things at home together in a long time. He's been hospitalized five times this year. He's been very oppositional and I can't do activities with him when he refuses to listen and go to school. I don't want to reward bad behavior. I did what I had to do like the shopping and the wash. Gary had to come along with me. He wanted to play Nintendo or do fun stuff with me during the day and on the weekend, but I did not allow it.

For Joseph and Teresa, the parent-child group provided an environment more conducive to productive activity than his room. When Teresa visited, she regularly brought *Highlights*, a children's magazine, puzzles, or a deck of cards. Teresa felt that it was important that their visits were productive and that they did things that would be educational or fun for Joseph.

> Joseph likes doing puzzles and it helps him calm down and focus. It's hard to do things with him on the unit because other children are there and always interrupting. It's hard for Joseph to settle down anyway to talk with me. There's a lot of important things that I want to talk about with him like how his day was, how he did in school and what level that he is on.

In the parent-child group, she and Joseph can leave the unit and go to an environment in which interactions are more controlled than they are visiting on the unit. The other children are involved with their parents so Teresa has an opportunity to help Joseph to focus and really work on something. "It's still hard for him to do anything because he can't focus or sit long. They better find the right medication for him."

As Joseph's hospitalization dragged into its third month, Teresa's frustration with Joseph's behavior was evident and her patience waned in the parent-child group. One evening she repeated that the doctors better regulate his medication better, but she added how horrible her grandson's behavior had been. "I haven't seen any changes. He had a terrible day at school and wasn't able to stay in class. He's been wild and unable to sit." Teresa said this on an evening when she had done most of the project that she and Joseph tried to do together. Joseph's movements when he attempted to participate in decorating a cardboard box with glue and glitter were fast and impulsive. He expressed anger each time that he attempted to participate. "Now, it's ruined! Throw it away!" He hid his head in his shirt and pulled away from the table. Each time, Teresa fixed the mistake to Joseph's satisfaction and he tried again to participate, only to repeat the sequence of interaction with his grandmother.

When it was time to go in the gym, Joseph raced ahead and got a large red ball with a diameter of approximately four feet from Ruth. When he brought it to his grandmother to play, Teresa exclaimed, "Bring that back! We are not going to play with that! It will make you too wild!" Joseph ran back to Ruth and this time took a paddle ball game. When he returned to Teresa, she said, "Now sit down and do a timeout to calm down." While Joseph walked over to a bench built into the gym wall and sat down to do a timeout, Teresa walked over to the next bench along the same wall to talk with Ruth. Joseph sat for a while with his head upside down and then he climbed up on the radiators, which were above the bench that he was sitting on. He banged his feet intermittently on the radiator. Teresa looked over and with frustration said to Ruth, "He's out of control and needs to go back to the unit. Call a nursing staff member to come and get him." Ruth called the unit and Joseph calmly walked back to the unit with a nursing staff member. Teresa said good night to Joseph and then continued talking with Ruth about her frustrations with Joseph.

The children similarly reported differences in their interactions with their parents in parent-child group from other interactions that they typically have.

Gary stated:

At home, we usually didn't do projects. We just played games sometimes, if my mother had the time. She didn't a lot because she always helps my brothers. I think that it's not fair for me. I have two brothers so she can't just play with me. I guess they have harder homework and I can do my homework by myself. I don't get time with her. When my mother visits when there's no parent-child group, it makes me sad. She always talks to me about being in the hospital and doing bad at home. I have to stop fighting with my brothers.

Another boy, Tom remarked: "It's fun making stuff with my father. My father was always busy at home. We never got to do that much." Joshua commented:

At home, I just like to watch videos and play videogames. I like to sit close and kiss my mother. We do that a lot. They don't like it when I do that here. Staff tells me to stop. Sometimes, I wrestle with Bob at home; I like to pin him on the floor. That's really fun. I can't do that here either.

The leaders report that the children act differently in parent-child group than they do in other groups or when they are going about their everyday activities on the unit. Beth noted:

Kids relax in the group; they're different than they are on the unit. Timmy was calling out and had a hard time staying on task. He was interrupting other kids and kind of anxious at times. He asked more than once, "When is my dad coming? When is he visiting?" So it's kind of like, "Thank God! We made it! We made it to this time."

Ruth's comments reflect a similar opinion. She said:

The children can be so focused unlike other groups. They are less hyper and act out less. When you see these kids in this group as opposed to on the unit or in other groups, they all seem to just kind of calm down, like the stress is taken off of them a little bit. They're off the unit with their families. You can see how comforting it is to them, even though they have these problems, they have these issues; you can see how they're so much more relaxed in the group.

Ruth elaborated on how the group seemed to open a door that led her to see children differently than she does in her everyday interactions with them on the inpatient unit.

> In parent-child group, I develop a special kind of affection for these kids because you see them in a different way. You see them more as unique children than you do when you work with them all day long on the unit like the nurses. On the unit, you get caught up getting the children to comply and follow the rules. When you take them out of that environment and put them in this group, you see the kid. When you come to parent-child group and see the kid in contact with their family, you see their life and you see the kids as opposed to whether they made level 2. You see them as part of a family, not just as mentally ill children.

I observed some negative cases of this theme. At times, parents told me that their children's behavior in the group was very similar to the behaviors that led to their hospitalization. For example, in the first group that Timmy attended, he tried to trip Mike, his father, by hooking a hockey stick around Mike's leg. Timmy laughed. In another group early in his hospitalization, after running around, Timmy sat on the floor and began to bang a hockey stick against his head. Mike reported that Timmy was self-abusive and regularly tried to hit or hurt him at home.

Joseph's mother Delia attended one parent-child group alone with Joseph and came to the next parent child group with Teresa, his grandmother. Teresa said that Joseph's explosive behavior during a basketball game with her and his mother was not unusual. Joseph became enraged when Teresa was taking basketball shots while he was tying his shoes. Later, he said that it was unfair that Teresa took shots while he was tying his shoes. Joseph has had attacks of rage since age three. She also noted that he especially became angry with her when his mother was present or immediately after a visit from her.

When Sam continuously lambasted his mother about her parenting and how he felt that she favored his foster brother, she commented that this was similar to his actions towards her at home. The only difference was that he didn't hit her at the hospital. Pat did her best to hide her feelings, but said, "I've come all the way up here for this? I can't take him home when he behaves like this."

We Connect

Before the group begins, some children appear very sad and parents struggle to interact with them. Sometimes the novelty of a new activity opens a door for a parent and child to have a playful interaction, which hasn't seemed possible recently or hasn't occurred for a long period of time. This brief connection in activity may be an open door to other positive interchanges:

> Christian looked sad and sullen at the beginning of group. He began crying and put his head on the table as he and his mother, Tara, tried to work on coloring a design. Though he stopped crying and was able to continue coloring after a leader took him for a short walk to the water fountain, his expression remained sullen. An occupational therapy student suggested that Christian and his mother try playing netball, a game, which they never played. Each player holds an individual small net with both hands; when the net is pulled taut, the ball pops up and can be caught by the other player. Tara said, "Let's see who can make the ball go higher." Christian was soon smiling and engaged in a friendly competition with his mother. A short while later, Christian asked for a basketball. He and Tara played basketball for the remainder of the group. There was eye contact and playfulness between mother and child.

> During his first night on the unit, 11-year-old Brian attended the parent-child group. He arrived teary-eyed with his head down. When the activity, sculpting animals using oven-baked putty, was introduced, he seemed to look past the leader. Though his parents and brother immediately took a piece of the Sculpey™ and began experimenting with it, he sat with his head down, although he periodically seemed to eye what they were doing. After a while, he picked up some clay and began shaping an animal with it. He looked brighter, worked intently and began talking with his parents about his project. After he made his first overtures of the night toward his mother, she drew closer to him and admired his work. A little later, I saw her assisting Brian in putting in the facial features of the male figure that he was making.

One parent's perception of a new connection to her child was not immediately evident to me. Tyrone's adoptive mother, Betty, a woman in her sixties, stated that the group provided her with opportunity to do something active with her son, which she didn't do at home. She described her interactions with Tyrone at home as typically negative; she yelled at him a great deal. In the first groups that she attended, I commented in my logs that she exhibited impatience and was curt with Tyrone when he did not immediately follow her task instructions. Though from my perspective as an outside observer, Betty's initiations and responses to Tyrone in those groups felt negative, Betty reported feeling good about her interactions; she reported that they were more positive than her interactions with Tyrone had been at home. Tyrone stated that he liked going to the parent-child group with his mother. In fact, on the day that he was discharged, he and Betty waited and attended the parent-child group before going home for good.

Another mother perceived growth one evening in her son's ability to interact with her and his sister while the leader did not perceive the events of that evening in the same way. From Ruth's point of view, 10-year-old Rasheem and his 12-year-old sister Dasia, had a terrible evening together as they worked on building a kite. They were argumentative. They pulled materials from one another's hands. Mrs. Brown, on the other hand, was very pleased that Rasheem participated in an activity with her and his sister. She said, "He's very difficult, you know. He will never sit down with us and do something with us as a family. Sure, he argued with Dasia, but he was working with her. He's never done that before in my recollection. It was a wonderful evening."

The following is an excerpt from my log on that evening:

> Rasheem's sister, Dasia, cut their piece of paper from the roll and then asked Rasheem to help her draw and then cut out the kite. He said, "NO!" He, at first, was insistent, but then helped a little. Dasia took charge and seemed to take ownership of this step of the task. After the kite was cut out, Rasheem said that it was bad and that they needed to redo it. It was too small. He pointed out the corners where Dasia cut off part of the corners. Ruth looked anxious, possibly at the thought that they might have to do it again. She said that they could fix it. They could add a piece to the side if they wanted. They needed to figure out how they wanted it to look. Rasheem looked up and said, "Do you think that this is Reading Rainbow?" He and his sister then refocused on the kite and went to work on fixing it. They added a small piece to each side and then Rasheem said, "That's good enough." Dasia agreed and then they looked for stencils so that they could decorate their kite. Dasia picked some and started to trace them.

Rasheem drifted off to the side. He seemed to lose interest. Mrs. Brown moved in close to Dasia as Dasia began tracing. Dasia remained very interested in the project. It may have been easier for Mrs. Brown to work with her as opposed to attempting to engage Rasheem. After a while, Ruth asked Rasheem to find a way to work with his mother and sister. Ruth suggested that Mrs. Brown sit in the middle, but that seating arrangement didn't work earlier in the group. After hearing Ruth's comment, Mrs. Brown called Rasheem to come over by her and help Dasia and her trace. At first, he said no, but then he came over and stood between Dasia and Mrs. Brown and took a turn tracing. In getting settled into the project, he and his sister jostled one another. Rasheem grabbed stencils and a pencil, which were in front of Dasia. Dasia grabbed them back and threatened to hit Rasheem if he didn't let go. Ruth intervened and told them to separate immediately. Rasheem ended up with the stencil and pencil, which he used to put one more design on the kite.

Beth suggested that Rasheem and Dasia take turns gluing and then putting glitter onto the areas that were stenciled. "No! I mess up the glue part. I get carried away with that stuff. I'll do all the glitter." Rasheem exclaimed. "No, you won't!" Dasia retorted. Beth told him that he could certainly take a turn putting the glue in the stencil area. If it was hard, Beth said that she was sure that his mother would help him. She then told him to stand near his mother as he did his gluing. Rasheem took his turn putting on the glue and appeared to do a fine enough job. He wasn't as attentive to detail as his sister, but the results were satisfactory to him, as well as to his sister. Rasheem tended to get carried away with the glitter; he dumped nearly a full 4-ounce container on one stencil. Dasia and his mother helped him dump the glitter off the page to limit how much glitter ended up on the table and floor.

Other times, there appears to be a wall of anger and great distance between a parent and child even though they may be standing or sitting next to each other. Some parents appeared to be openly rejecting overtures from their children or ignoring them. A new engaging activity that brought out playfulness in both parent and child sometimes changed the mood. Below is an example from my logs about an evening of interaction between Jason and his mother, Sally.

When they went to the gym, Jason told his mother, Sally, that he wanted to play basketball. With disdain, Sally said that she wasn't playing that game. Jason whined and begged a little and attempting to compromise, said that they could just shoot and stand in one spot. "Absolutely not!" Sally retorted. Beth explained that parent-child group was about finding activities that both a parent and a child could enjoy doing together, not just an activity that a child could do with anyone at some other time. She showed them how to play with the large elastic badminton paddles and birdie. Sally's eyes brightened a little as they started to play. Jason also became more animated about playing the game with his mother. You could hear laughter and they both stayed focused on each other while they played the game for about ten minutes. This was in sharp contrast to what occurred during the structured activity. Earlier they worked on crafts side by side with little conversation. Sally was very short with Jason and jumped on comments that he made. "What are you making?" Jason asked. "WHAT DOES IT LOOK LIKE!" Sally sarcastically answered.

Over the course of attending parent-child activity group, a parent and child participate in a tabletop or physical activity. They may become reacquainted with each other and find a way to connect with each other in an activity that they haven't found before. Tom's interactions with his father are an example of this.

Tom was hospitalized three times this year. During his first two hospitalizations, his mother visited him regularly and participated in the parent-child group with him. His father periodically attended the parent-child group with his wife and son, but he sat back and quietly watched his wife and son work together. When Tom gave his mother a hard time about how a project was turning out or resisted her overtures to help, his father did not react or participate in the interaction. Christine, one of the leaders, felt that Mrs. Boland held in a great deal of anger with Mr. Boland though she acted sweetly in public. Mrs. Boland reported that at home, Mr. Boland worked a great deal and when he wasn't working, he kept his distance from Tom and left her most often to deal with Tom's behavior outbursts. Christine decided that the parent-child group would be a good place to get Mr. Boland to interact more with Tom. Having Mr. and Mrs. Boland in the group with Tom at the same time wasn't working, so she planned to invite Mr. Boland to come to group alone with Tom.

The project was in front of Tom; initially his father quietly helped placing puzzle pieces on the frame; Tom picked out the puzzle pieces from the bucket and seemed in charge of the activity. There seemed to be a good working relationship around doing the picture frame between Tom and his father. Mr. Boland seemed to be following Tom's cues. There was minimal conversation between them; they quietly worked. As they got further into the project, they began to experiment with the pieces especially around doing a person for the inside of the frame. They laughed and talked about what to use for a hat; Tom hunted for little beads in the bucket for arms. They tried one piece for a goatee for the man. Tom said that he didn't like it; his father gently directed him to try another piece. After Tom found another piece to use for a beard, he looked down at his project and then glanced at his father with a smile saying; "Now that looks good!"

Mr. Boland asked Tom for a piece and shaped a dog; he smiled and told Tom to check it out. Tom smiled and said now watch this, "Now it is a dog laying down in the street and now it is a dog smashed by a car." The clay was now smashed. Mr. Boland rolled his eyes and then said, "Come on. Let's make something else." Tom said, "No, wait a minute, the dog needs tire tracks all over him." Mr. Boland smiled, but shook his head and kneaded the clay and gave Tom some. Tom said, "Let's make a rabbit." He got busy and focused on shaping a rabbit. Mr. Boland had a little piece and made a small animal. Tom looked up after a while, smiled at his dad, then laughed and said "Dad, what's that? Are you making a rat?" The Mr. Boland looked back at him smiled and said that he didn't know; he made a tail and then made an animal to go with the tail. The overall impression that I felt from watching Tom and his dad is that they enjoy being together in the group. They made a lot of eye contact, sat side by side, smiled at each other, talked and worked at a relaxed pace.

At the end of Tom's hospitalization, Christine commented to Tom and Mr. Boland:

You know, it was amazing to watch you guys do things together. It looked like you really had a good time together in group. I hope that you continue this. You know, find some time every day to sit down and do something together. I think that would really help Tom.

Some parents also make connections about their own interactions with their children while watching and listening to interactions between other parents and children in the group.

As Tom and his father worked on a picture frame, Christine talked with Jenny and her family about how Jenny and her sisters provoked one another and how with the back and forth of challenges and threats, no child was innocent. After group, Mr. Boland stopped to talk to Christine. Mr. Boland said, "You know, I kind of realized that what you were talking about with Jenny's family happens at my house too. I said to Tom, 'You know, it's not all you, your brother has a responsibility for the way things go back and forth ping pong style. I know it's not all your fault. I will do a much better job at being aware of how things go back and forth and how I can put a stop to it. But to do that, I need your commitment that you can help me put a stop to it.'

On a different note, Kathy reported understanding and supporting the goals of the group, and regularly attended, but did not expect her child to participate in the activity. In the first two groups that Kathy and Joshua attended, Kathy talked about encouraging Joshua to participate more, but she retreated from that plan and did a great deal of the projects herself. The projects reflected her preferences as opposed to Joshua's. Kathy made excuses for Joshua's limited involvement such as Joshua being tired and not liking arts and crafts. Though Kathy began to take the lead in the third group that they attended, Joshua was active and clear about what he wanted to do that evening and how he wanted his dinosaur project to look. She reported being surprised at Joshua's increased engagement in activity, backed off and allowed Joshua to take over his own activity. Joshua watched other boys work on projects with their parents and talk among themselves; he worked his way into the conversation of two boys about wrestling and dinosaurs. After this group, Kathy stated that she saw hope that Joshua would be able to have friends and participate in group activities like other children do.

Parents' attitudes toward the children seemed to be an important factor relative to whether parents used the group to engage their children as described in this chapter. Some caregivers such as Mike, Teresa, and Andrea, persisted in attending group and in attempting to engage their children in spite of the children's inattention, aggressiveness, or intermittent resistance to their initiations. They accepted the notion that the group was about sharing an activity with their children and worked toward that goal. They did not retaliate in the group when their children resisted their attempts to engage them. The parents who experienced the group as positive may have been more motivated for participation, had more hope, developed stronger connections with the leaders or with me as a researcher. They may have experienced less family or life stress, or have had less troubled relationships with their children than those parents who did not appear to experience the group as positive or particularly productive. In spite of these possible differences, it is instructive to reflect upon what I observed occurring in parent-child group for those caregivers and children for whom the group seemed less helpful.

A CONVERSATION:
RESEARCH QUESTIONS, FINDINGS AND LITERATURE

The struggles and problems that parents in this study reported about their interactions with their children, parallel reports in the literature about family interaction when children exhibit mental illness (Crowell, Feldman & Ginsberg, 1988; Dumas, 1996; Field et al., 1987; Johnston, 1996; Preston, 1990). One mother stated that she often yelled at her son and never played with him. Four parents described being physically harmed by their children on a regular basis. Most described instances of their children's violent temper tantrums at home and in public. These reports are also consistent with the literature on family burden and grief related to taking care of a family member with mental illness. Though I did not ask parents about the burden of caring for their children, many parents with whom I spoke spontaneously shared stories about the trials of living with their children. The experiences that the caregivers described about caring for their children with mental illness seem similar to reports about the burden of caring for adult family members with mental illness (Jeon & Madjar, 1998; Pickett, Cook, & Cohler, 1994; Scazufca & Kuipers, 1998; Solomon & Draine, 1996).

Difficulties managing the symptoms of their children's mental illness colored the daily activity interactions between parents and their offspring. Andrea described how Gary and one of her other sons fought violently with each other and didn't respond to her directions or limits. She said that she didn't want to reward negative behavior by participating in enjoyable activities with them. Kathy said that she didn't dare disturb Joshua as he watched videos because she expected a temper tantrum. She felt the need to bathe Joshua because she felt that he was not able to adequately complete this self-care activity without her assistance. Mike similarly reported providing physical care for Matthew as his symptoms of mental illness increased.

Parental expectations of conflict with their children also had a significant impact on how the parents interacted with their psychiatrically hospitalized children. Mike and Mr. Mendez, Carlos' father, stated that they expected their sons to ruin family outings by having temper tantrums. Both fathers described themselves as being held hostage in their homes because of their sons' typical aggressive behavior. Mike talked extensively about how he anticipated trouble and how he attempted to head off the trouble by controlling his child's environment or altering his own behavior. These expectations influenced how the parents reacted to their children while they were hospitalized. One interaction between Rasheem and his mother, Ms. Brown, graphically illustrated this point. As parents turned to leave the child inpatient unit after the parent-child group, Rasheem ran down the long hall of the unit toward the opened back door. Ms. Brown was standing by the open door talking to a group leader when she saw Rasheem racing toward the door. Her body stiffened and she shouted, "No! Stop!" Rasheem continued to run until he reached her and looked confused. He said that he had forgotten to kiss her good night. When Ms. Brown realized his intentions, she relaxed as much as she could and hugged her son.

In spite of initial negative expectations of their children's behaviors, parents reported having positive experiences with their children in the parent-child activity group. These findings are similar to the report by Alexander, Barton, Waldron, and Mas (1989) in which they found that when a positive focus on verbal interaction was facilitated, family members were less accusatory of each other than when they discussed problem behaviors. In the present study, parents and children most often reported feeling positive about the group and talked about enjoying their time together. This contrasts with their reports about having limited, unpleasant, or difficult experiences in their daily interaction with each other prior to the hospitalization, or about being dissatisfied with the quality of their interaction on the inpatient unit. Alexander, Barton, Waldron, and Mas (1989) stated that the positive effect on family interactions in their study did not last after the families were allowed to interact in typical negative ways, but suggested that repeated opportunities to interact in a positive context might lead to a lasting change in how families interact.

In this research study, it was observed that after families had participated in the parent-child group over a few weeks and had repeated positive experiences, some families exhibited change within the context of the group. Mike, Timmy's father, reported enjoying activities with his son that he did not enjoy when he entered the group at the beginning of Timmy's hospitalization. He also reported successful attempts to engage Timmy in activity when they left the hospital grounds together. According to Beth, one of the group leaders, both Joseph and Gary began to approach activities with their parents in a more active and positive way over the course of their multiple hospitalizations. The leaders and caregivers reported that during their first hospitalizations, neither child actively participated in parent-child activity. They withdrew at minimal challenge and left Teresa and Andrea to complete the projects on their own. Jason and Rasheem had periods of positive activity engagement with their mothers during their brief sojourns in the parent-child group. Though those moments felt hopeful to me as a participant observer, I do not know if their experiences in the group had an impact on how these parents and children interacted outside of the group.

REFERENCES

Alexander, J. F., Waldron, H. B., Barton, C., & Mas, C. H. (1989). The minimizing of blaming attributions and behaviors in delinquent families. *Journal of Consulting and Clinical Psychology, 57*, 19-24.

Bogdan, R. C., & Biklen, S. K. (1992). *Qualitative research for education: An introduction to theory and methods* (2nd ed.). Boston, MA: Allyn and Bacon.

Crowell, J. A., Feldman, S. S., & Ginsberg, N. (1988). Assessment of mother-child interaction in preschoolers with behavior problems. *Journal of the Academy of Child and Adolescent Psychiatry, 27*, 303-311.

Denzin, N. K., & Lincoln, Y. S. (Eds.). (1994). *Handbook of qualitative research.* Thousand Oaks, CA: Sage.

Dumas, J. E. (1996). Why was this child referred? Interaction correlates of referral status in families of children with disruptive behavior problems. *Journal of Clinical Child Psychology, 25*, 106-115.

Ely, M., Anzul, M., Friedman, T., Garner, D., & Steinmetz, A. M. (1991). *Doing qualitative research: Circles within circles.* London: The Falmer Press.

Ely, M., Vinz, R., Downing, M., & Anzul, M. (1997). *On writing qualitative research: Living by words.* London: The Falmer Press.

Field, T., M., Sandberg, D., Goldstein, S., Garcia, R., Vega-Lahr, N., Porter, K., & Dowling, M. (1987). Play interactions and interviews of depressed and conduct disorder children and their mothers. *Child Psychiatry and Human Development, 17,* 213-234.

Fontana, A., & Frey, J. H. (1994). Interviewing: The art of science. In N. K. Denzin & Y. S. Lincoln (Eds.), *Handbook of qualitative research* (pp. 361-376). Thousand Oaks, CA: Sage Publications, Inc.

Jeon, Y. & Madjar, I. (1998). Caring for a family member with chronic mental illness. *Qualitative Health Research, 8,* 694-706.

Johnston, C. (1996). Parent characteristics and parent-child interactions in families of nonproblem children and ADHD children with higher and lower levels of oppositional-defiant behavior. *Journal of Abnormal Child Psychology, 24,* 85-104.

Lincoln,Y. S., & Guba, E. G. (1985). *Naturalistic inquiry.* Beverly Hills, CA: Sage.

Lofland, J., & Lofland, L. (1984). *Analyzing social settings: A guide to qualitative observation and analysis* (2nd. Ed.). Belmont, CA: Wadsworth.

Pickett, S. A., Cook, J. A., & Cohler, B. J. (1994). Caregiving burden experienced by parents of offspring with severe mental illness: The impact of off-timedness. *Journal of Applied Social Sciences, 18,* 199-207.

Preston, T. (1990). Parents' perceptions of behavior in disturbed children: A study of attributions, affect, and expectancies. (Doctoral dissertation, Vanderbilt University, 1990). *Dissertation Abstracts International, 51,* (5-B) 2632.

Scazufca, M. & Kuipers, E. (1998). Stability of expressed emotion in relatives of those with schizophrenia and its relationship with burden of care and perception of patients' social functioning. *Psychological Medicine, 28,* 453-461.

Solomon, P. & Draine, J. (1996). Examination of grief among family members of individuals with serious and persistent mental illness. *Psychiatric Quarterly, 67,* 221-234.

doi:10.1300/J004v22n03_05

Chapter 6

Exploring What Was Missing
in One Parent-Child Activity Group

SUMMARY. Barriers to parent-child interaction that arose in the parent-child activity group studied by the author are discussed. An analysis of what factors within the group may have led to the barriers is
provided so that readers can consider how to minimize barriers to parent-
child interaction in similar groups. doi:10.1300/J004v22n03_06 *[Article
copies available for a fee from The Haworth Document Delivery Service:
1-800-HAWORTH. E-mail address: <docdelivery@haworthpress.com> Website:
<http://www.HaworthPress.com> © 2006 by The Haworth Press, Inc. All rights
reserved.]*

KEYWORDS. Parent-child activity groups, parent-child interaction,
group environment

In addition to finding ways that the parent-child activity group appeared to open doors for interaction between caregivers and children
within my qualitative research data, I also came to see parent-child
interactional barriers in the way that the group was led. As a researcher

[Haworth co-indexing entry note]: "Exploring What Was Missing in One Parent-Child Activity
Group." Olson, Laurette. Co-published simultaneously in *Occupational Therapy in Mental Health* (The
Haworth Press, Inc.) Vol. 22, No. 3/4, 2006, pp. 83-101; and: *Activity Groups in Family-Centered Treat-
ment: Psychiatric Occupational Therapy Approaches for Parents and Children* (Laurette Olson) The
Haworth Press, Inc., 2006, pp. 83-101. Single or multiple copies of this article are available for a fee from
The Haworth Document Delivery Service [1-800- HAWORTH, 9:00 a.m. - 5:00 p.m. (EST). E-mail ad-
dress: docdelivery@haworthpress.com].

and a therapist, it is important to examine what appeared to work as well as what didn't appear to work for families. Critically thinking about how one intervenes with clients allows clinicians to learn from experience and improve their capacities as helping professionals (Gambrill, 1990; Evans, 2001). New ways of looking at what occurred in the parent-child activity group may be discovered which in turn may lead to reconsideration of approaches to helping families.

As I clustered my codes and developed categories in the course of my data analysis, I noted that I had categories of concerns about how some elements of the group appeared to limit interactions between parents and children. In my final analysis, I placed these categories in this metatheme, "Barriers are blocking the door." I have worked to present each barrier with vignettes from my participant observation so that readers can reflect upon them and consider my analysis in relation to them. Within this discussion of barriers, I have also shared 4 incidents when I left my role as a researcher because I felt that what was occurring or about to occur would be harmful to parents' and children's abilities to interact with one another in the group. This is important because it allows readers to have some understanding about how my experience as the developer and a leader of a parent-child activity group challenged my role as a researcher. I may have had more insight into the needs of parents and children within a parent-child activity group than I might have had without my experience, but my experience also brought up ethical concerns that I felt required action. I present this to readers to consider along with my analysis. Who I am as a clinician is as present in this chapter as who I am as the researcher of this study.

The barriers that stood out to me most as I analyzed my data were related to the activities that the leaders chose to introduce to families, how participants were seated relative to one another at the activities table, and how leaders conversed or didn't converse with parents and children. As I wrote this chapter, I saw an additional barrier, the influence of Managed Care on child psychiatric treatment and the parent-child activity group. This chapter will be divided into four subsections that identify and describe each barrier.

THE ACTIVITIES:
SOMETIMES THEY DON'T HELP US INTERACT

Beth and Ruth, two group leaders, believed that parents and children would change their interaction styles if given the opportunity to participate in arts and crafts and gross motor activities in a neutral and structured environment. They expected parents and children to listen to leader requests for each family to work and play as a unit during the group. Both Beth and Ruth commented about how frustrating it was that some parents and children didn't interact around the activities even when reminded.

Beth and Ruth chose the arts and crafts and the gross motor activities when they led the group. They chose one arts and crafts activity per group and provided all of the necessary supplies. All participating families would individually complete that project. When the craft activity was complete, families were directed to straighten up their work area and move into the gym. In the gym, they provided the gross motor equipment that children requested. The requests were typically for basketballs and floor hockey equipment. They rarely made suggestions of alternative activities to parents and children, even when some mothers were inappropriately attired, for example by wearing high heels, the children were overly active or aggressive, or the children intended to play an active sport with elderly or apparently exhausted caregivers.

Christine and Maria, two other group leaders, acquiesced to Beth or Ruth with regard to the activity choice and materials. Christine often asked families to focus the arts and crafts activity on expressing something about their families. For example, when creating a book was the activity, Christine asked that families create a book of the activities that family members enjoy doing together.

Beth reported that she had a range of activities and craft supplies readily available in the group room and quickly chose an activity for each group. She said that she tended to use the same cycle of activities because children's hospitalizations tend to be short and families usually attended the group only a few times. Beth did not report any particular plan for choosing activities other than choosing those that she felt would interest the children on the unit in general because she was never sure who would attend the group on a particular night. Ruth reported choosing activities the same way.

Often, activities that I observed in the parent-child group didn't require interaction between parents and children. The activities, such as coloring or making cards, were most often simple enough for a child to do alone or the prepared materials were not big enough for two sets of hands to touch without conflict. In spite of this, Ruth told me after groups where she introduced such activities that she was trying to get families to work together. After group one evening, she expressed a great deal of frustration with Joseph's grandmother, Teresa, because Teresa took her own coloring project and colored parallel to Joseph. Each page to be colored was approximately 5 by 8 inches.

When parents and children worked parallel to each other, there was little or no conversation. Sometimes, conversation seemed to intrude or interfere with solitary activity, as occurred between Jason and his mother, Sally.

> Jason, a nine-year-old boy, quietly worked on making a birthday card for his uncle. His mother, Sally, sat next to him working on her own card for the uncle. "What are you making?" Jason asks. "What does it look like!" she sarcastically retorted. "It looks like one of those tattoos." "Well, it's not!" His mother seems emotionally cold and distant and primarily interested in doing her own card.

Some activities could be done piecemeal and didn't provoke emotion or seem particularly meaningful to either parent or child. Participants seemed just to be getting through the activity.

> Carlos sat throughout the group looking into the distance out the window. He intermittently completed part of a task only when his mother insisted and then he quickly drifted out of the activity. Mrs. Mendez worked diligently to give Carlos tasks to do, but she approached engaging Carlos as a supervisor on an assembly line. She assigned Carlos jobs related to the project, but she and Carlos hadn't worked out a plan for their joint project. They hadn't discussed what he wanted the project to look like or what he was interested in doing. They were copying the leaders' model.

Beth frequently attempted to cajole children into participation. She changed activities for some of the children who resisted participation, but she didn't include parents in the decision to change the activity. For example, when Gary was resistive to participating in the activities presented in the parent-child group one evening, Beth brought out a wooden car. She told Gary that she thought he might like to paint it. He smiled and said that he would like to paint it. He worked on painting the car over two group sessions. The activity interested Gary and he participated in the solitary activity of painting the car over the next two sessions, but his mother was left to watch.

On three occasions, I left my role as participant observer when I felt that the activity structure was particularly destructive to the parents' and children's ability to interact. One evening, Ruth had given Rasheem an ultimatum about doing a particular project or losing gym time. Rasheem and Ruth's interaction was quickly developing into a power struggle; Rasheem's mother and sister watched as outsiders. Rasheem was not going to back down and would likely be sent back to the unit for non-compliance and for speaking rudely to Ruth. If this occurred, Rasheem, his mother, and his sister would lose the opportunity to interact that evening. Below is an excerpt from my field log about how I recorded the interchange, including how I briefly stepped out of my researcher's role to intervene.

> Rasheem said that he didn't like to color and didn't like the dinosaur puzzle that Ruth put out for children to color this evening. Ruth said that he would have to do it if he wanted to go into the gym. Ruth did not try to engage him in the activity or try to change the activity to engage him. I could only think of one way to help Ruth and Rasheem within the constraints that Ruth had created. Since Rasheem left an opener by saying that he did not like dinosaurs and had talked about liking baseball, I asked him about making a baseball picture for the puzzle. I suggested that he turn the puzzle over and make a picture that he liked. Both Ruth and Rasheem seemed to like the idea.

This seemed to provide Rasheem with a way to save face. He did not give in; he accepted an alternative. From Ruth's perspective, Rasheem complied with her demand to participate in the activity that she had provided. Participating in the activity was still challenging for Rasheem, but his mother and sister were able to respond to his specific frustrations with it. Below is what happened next.

> Rasheem said that he wanted to write METS in bubble letters but didn't know how to do it. His sister offered to write the letters for him, Rasheem then drew a baseball; his mother added a bat to the picture. Rasheem demanded that his mother color the picture. He colored with his mother's coaxing although he intermittently said that he wasn't doing any more because his picture wasn't coming out right. He leaned on his mother in between demanding that she do it and coloring himself; his mother stroked his head and coaxed him to color more; he complied with each request.

On another evening, Sara, an occupational therapy student, led the group using a lesson plan for making butterflies. There is a definite right and wrong way to complete this kind of close-ended project. This set Sara up as an expert and she then responded in kind to all requests for help. When one five-year-old child asked for scissors, Sara became engaged in teaching the child to cut and structuring the activity so that he could cut. She neglected to include the child's mother, Ms. Johnson, who had previously been trying to help her child with his project. Ms. Johnson, a young mother who seemed tentative about her ability to assist her very active son, typically persisted when she attempted to help him complete a task in parent-child activity group. On this occasion, she shrunk into the background and did not give any sign of challenging Sara's intrusion. After observing for a few minutes, I redirected Sara to let Ms. Johnson hold the scissors for her son, Billy, and told Ms. Johnson that she should help Billy cut. I moved the project from between Sara and Billy to between Billy and his mother. I asked Sara to provide guide Ms. Johnson as necessary in teaching her son to cut.

I also observed an occupational therapy student, Martha, who unwittingly excluded a set of parents from an activity that parents typically relish doing for their children–presenting a birthday cake. Mr. and Mrs. Connor brought a birthday cake for their son, Lee, on the evening of the group. They planned to stay and enjoy the cake with their son and other children on the unit, but decided to join the group when Martha said that they could share the cake at the end of the session. Martha took the cake from them when they arrived in the group room and put it in the small supply room in the back.

Halfway through the group, Martha noted that families were very involved in their projects and were working at a slower pace than usual. Martha disappeared into the back supply room. When I glanced over I saw that she was lighting the cake. I walked to the back to find out her plan for the birthday cake. Martha said that she decided to serve the cake while the families were busy painting. She had decided that the participants could eat a slice of cake while they worked. In this way, Martha said she thought the group would move along routinely and end on time. She planned to do this without consulting the parents who brought the cake. It also felt to me that Martha had taken ownership of the cake as a hostess might when a guest brings a cake to a dinner party.

Since there was no leader present, I stepped out of my role as a researcher and directed Martha to take the candles out of the cake and to leave the cake where it was. We then waited until all of the participants finished their projects and cleaned up their work area. Then Martha helped the participants set the table while Lee's parents went into the back supply room to light their son's birthday cake. Both the parents and the child smiled broadly throughout the process of the parents bringing in the cake, and enjoyed themselves during the singing and their sharing of the cake with all of the participants of the group that evening.

Joseph and his grandmother Teresa's experiences were different from those of other families because Joseph's present hospitalization was much longer than the other children's hospitalization. In addition, this was his second hospitalization during this study. Teresa was very invested in the parent-child group throughout Joseph's two hospitalizations. In the beginning of Joseph's second hospitalization during this study, she attended two groups in one week even though she traveled over an hour to get to the hospital. Beth reported that Teresa and Joseph were regular group members during his previous hospitalizations, as well. Towards the end of Joseph's last hospitalization, Teresa expressed increasing frustration and anger that the doctors were not able to find a medication to help Joseph better attend to tasks and control his aggressive and impulsive behavior. Both Joseph and Teresa understood that the purpose of this last hospitalization was to find a new medication that would not cause heart irregularities. Medical staff was now recommending residential care because they believed that Joseph's behavior issues were intractable and could not be managed at home. They were not hopeful that they would find a medication that would allow Joseph to return to Teresa's home or to succeed in a day hospital program. In addition, Teresa's daughter, Delia, who is Joseph's biological mother, began to visit Joseph after many months of not visiting him. Teresa reported that when Joseph had contact with Delia, he typically expressed more verbal and physical rage toward Teresa. Joseph's and Teresa's interaction in the parent-child group became increasingly tense. Joseph was less attentive and more impulsive; Teresa exhibited less patience. The following vignette occurred during this period of their group involvement.

When it was time to go in the gym, Joseph raced ahead and got a large red ball with a diameter of approximately 4 feet. When he brought it to his grandmother to play, Teresa exclaimed, "Bring that back! We are not going to play with that! It will make you too wild!" Joseph ran back to Ruth and this time took a paddle ball game. When he returned to Teresa, she said, "Now sit down and do a timeout to calm down." While Joseph walked over to a bench built into the gym wall and sat down to do a timeout, Teresa walked over to the next bench along the same wall to talk with Ruth. Joseph sat for a while with his head upside down and then he climbed up on the radiators above the bench. He banged his feet intermittently on the radiator. Teresa looked over with frustration and said, "He's out of control and needs to go back to the unit. Call a nursing staff member to come and get him!" Ruth called the unit and Joseph calmly walked back to the unit with a nursing staff member. Teresa said good night to Joseph and then continued talking with Ruth about her frustrations with Joseph.

As a researcher, I wrote a field log describing what occurred and also wrote about the how each participant may have viewed the incident differently. Ruth felt that Teresa needed someone to listen to her concerns about Joseph and to support her when she set a limit with him. Both she and Beth reported to me that they felt that Teresa didn't always set firm limits with Joseph when he exhibited uncontrolled behavior. Tonight, she did. Teresa's growing frustration with the course of Joseph's medical treatment was becoming overwhelming. Her patience was noticeably reduced and she appeared to have no energy for playing ball with Joseph as she had in the past. Joseph was having a hard time modulating his behavior in the large and distracting environment of the gymnasium. One perspective about Joseph's banging feet and head hanging upside down may be that these were signs of his continuing inability to control his physical behavior. Another perspective is that Joseph was growing impatient with the extended conversation between Ruth and his grandmother and was attempting to remind them of his presence.

On another evening, Joseph played basketball with Delia and Teresa. Within a short amount of time, Joseph became infuriated and screamed, "My grandmother cheats; she's shooting while I'm tying my shoes! I hate her!" After this outburst, Joseph ran to the front of the gym, and paced back and forth. A childcare worker was called and Joseph was escorted back to the inpatient unit without his mother and grandmother.

In this instance, the leaders observed and reacted to the outburst with safety in mind. Before the group, both Beth and Ruth commented to me that they expected that Joseph might have difficulty in the group because his mother was visiting along with his grandmother. From my perspective as an observer, I wondered whether the leaders could have prevented Joseph's outburst by introducing a less competitive and a more sedate activity than basketball. This might have helped Joseph have a calmer and more benign interaction with his mother and grand-mother than he had.

THE ODD CHILD OUT: PAY ATTENTION TO ME!

Some caregivers brought other children from the family to the par-ent-child group. At times, it was evident that these other children had a stronger relationship with the caregivers than the hospitalized children. At times, the non-hospitalized children sat between the caregivers and the hospitalized children, effectively reducing the possibilities for inter-action between them. Observations related to such seating arrange-ments and the subsequent exclusion of hospitalized children from family interaction was particularly striking and poignant to me.

Three examples highlight this point. Sometimes children did partici-pate in a project parallel to their caregivers, remained calm, and were task-focused throughout the group as was expected. Angry or sad feel-ings were expressed after the group ended. Other times, as in Walter's case, a child was unable to remain focused on the arts and crafts project.

Desiree attended group tonight with her grandmother, Ms. Smith, and her eight-year-old sister, Tanya. They sat in a line at the table with Tanya in the middle. Ms. Smith sat unoccupied and looked around most of the night. Periodically, Tanya asked Ms. Smith for help, which Ms. Smith readily provided. Ms. Smith's expression softened as she leaned over to help and speak with Tanya. She asked Tanya about her project and told her how well it was coming out. Desiree worked silently and sullenly on her project alone and without any interaction with her grandmother. Over the course of the evening, her grandmother rarely looked over at her. When her grandmother did, she appeared tense. At the end of the night, Ms. Smith and Tanya said good night to Desiree. Desiree quickly and respectfully kissed her grandmother on the cheek without making any other physical contact. Ms. Smith allowed the kiss, but didn't reciprocate or move closer to Desiree. She told Desiree that she would be back on the weekend. Desiree darted onto the unit. As the door closed behind her, she began sobbing loudly and uncon-trollably. Since I was the only adult in the area, I sat down with Desiree and comforted her for a few moments. I called Beth over to sit with Desiree and me on the couch. In between the tears and

Beth's comforting words and hugs, Desiree said that she didn't get to spend enough time with her grandmother. Beth asked her if she wanted help to talk to her grandmother more as she worked on her projects in group. Desiree nodded yes. Unfortunately, Ms. Smith never attended parent-child group again during Desiree's hospitalization.

Jorge worked side by side with Julia, his 22-year-old aunt and her five-year-old son. Julia recently adopted Jorge after the death of his grandmother, who had been his custodial parent. Julia sat close to her son and helped him make a dog with the modeling clay. Though Jorge sat next to them, he might have been sitting tables apart or in another room. There was no conversation or eye contact between him and Julia. Jorge periodically gazed over at Mr. Mendez, Carlos' father. Mr. Mendez was sculpting zoo animals with animation and flair while Carlos and his mother passively looked on. Jorge's smile broadened when he made eye contact with Mr. Mendez. Jorge made comments like, "I like that!" He imitated Mr. Mendez's technique and periodically Mr. Mendez offered him pointers. In the gym, Jorge played basketball alone while his Aunt Julia cuddled her son on the sideline.

At the end of the group, Jorge lined up next to his aunt and cousin as he was directed to. He and Julia had what appeared to be their first real conversation of the evening. Jorge apparently asked her when he was going home. He stormed off the line and cried out, "You love your son! Not ME!"

"I think *Walter* should go back to the unit now. He's not listening. He's up from the table and when I tell him to go back, he's mouthing off," Ruth called across the table to Beth. Laticia, Walter's mother, didn't look up. Walter sat two seats away from her. Darvon, Walter's four-year-old brother, sat between Laticia and Walter. Throughout the group, Laticia worked quietly on a project with Darvon while Walter worked alone.

CONVERSATION: WE NEED HELP TO TALK TOGETHER

During Sam's second and third hospitalization, he was openly resistive to participating in activities with his mother. He verbalized anger and resentment at her for hospitalizing him and for favoring his foster brother. Pat, his mother, was unable to respond effectively to Sam to end verbal assaults. Pat stopped attending parent-child group after the following experience.

At the start of one group, Sam was yelling at his mother about how the problems that led to his hospitalization were hers and not his. Pat looked down and softly said that Sam's behavior had to change if she was going to take home. Beth took Sam outside of the group room to talk and to calm down. Pat remained at the table. While she sat there, she commented to me, "I've come all the way up here for this? I can't take him home when he behaves like this. The only difference in his behavior here than it was at home, is that he can't hit me here. He will hit me again if he comes home like this."

Beth reported to me that she felt that Sam needed to calm down so she removed him from the room and she hoped that after she talked with him that he would be less verbally abusive to his mother. Sam calmed down after talking with Beth and was able to return to the group table, but his emotional reaction to his mother did not change. Sam was aligned with Beth; Pat remained an outsider and Sam's nemesis. Once seated next to his mother again, he returned to telling her off.

I observed that when children interacted in ways that parents seemed to experience as inappropriate, parents tended to look toward Beth to limit set or redirect the conversation as opposed to dealing with their children's behavior themselves. When Beth responded, she intervened directly with the children.

"What happened to your earring? You had one last week." Rasheem asked Joseph. Joseph shrugged and said that he didn't know; he just wasn't wearing it. Rasheem said that he would pull it out of Joseph's ear if Joseph wore it. He said that he was mad at Joseph the other day when they were in the gym playing basketball. Joseph didn't respond. A little bit later, Joseph said that he wanted to beat up another kid. Rasheem described how he messed up a kid before he came to the hospital. No adult said anything. Parents seemed uncomfortable with the conversation; Rasheem's mother looked down and shook her head in disapproval, and Joseph's grandmother widened her eyes and tensed her lips but looked toward Beth. Beth finally said, "I don't think that this is an appropriate conversation. Let's talk about something else."

Beth also initiated conversation with children. The conversation tended to remain a dialogue between her and the children as opposed to expanding to include parents.

Beth brought up Halloween and said that there would be a Halloween party next week. Rasheem said that he remembered it from the
last time that he was hospitalized. Joseph brought up that he
wanted to be Puppet Master, and Rasheem brought up some
equally violent and gruesome characters. Beth said that they both
knew that they couldn't be anything like that; that Halloween on
the unit is supposed to be fun and not too scary. They both kept on
naming scary characters that they would like to be. Rasheem said
that he was going to get out by Halloween "by keeping his behavior together." Joseph said that he would like to be Freddy Krueger
or Jason. Beth said that he knew better than to think that he could
be a scary character like that on Halloween. She said that she knew
he could come up with a more appropriate idea for a Halloween
costume. As she talked they both interrupted her with their ideas
for Halloween; as one spoke, the other seemed to increase in the
loudness and intensity of their speech. Beth said that she didn't
like their behavior and that her feelings were hurt when they interrupted her. She asked how they would feel if they were her. They
both stopped and apologized; she said that she didn't want just
words; she wanted their actions to show that they cared when she
spoke.

Though Beth successfully initiated or redirected the children's conversation, the parents were passive during these exchanges and did not
share their thoughts with their children. In reflecting upon what I observed and thinking about it relative to my own experiences as a leader,
I wondered whether Beth might have tried to talk with the parents about
her views of the situation and suggested ways of managing the children
or redirecting the conversation. At the same time, she might have also
engaged the children who may have been interested in what the adults
were talking about and in what the adults would decide. An interesting
conversation among parents and children may have been facilitated.
    Another way of looking at this vignette is to consider how culture
may have influenced how the children, parents and leaders behaved.
The leaders were white, middle class women, while the children and
caregivers participating in the interchange described were African
American and poor. Beth's expectations for conversation were that it be
a controlled and non-controversial exchange. The boys were comfortable with a fast, animated banter and sharing all of their thoughts including those that were shocking or confrontational. African-American
interpersonal dialogue has been described as "high-keyed, animated,

heated, and confrontational" while the interactional style of persons of a white, middle class background has been characterized as "detached, objective, and nonchallenging" (Sue & Sue, 1990, p. 64). The parents may have been sensitive to cultural clash and embarrassed by the boys' conversation as opposed to disapproving of it in the same way as Beth did.

In some instances, parents were observed to have what I consider inappropriate interactions with their children. For example, Ms. Reed was often observed to be openly negative and critical of her son, Devon. The interaction with his mother also seemed to be difficult for Devon. The group leaders, Ruth and Beth, did not intervene but simply watched. They privately commented to me later that Ms. Reed was defensive and was quick to criticize them as well. When she overheard them talking about ordering dinosaur projects for boys and flower projects for girls, Ms. Reed called them sexist. Their personal feelings about Ms. Reed seemed to have influenced their decision to distance themselves from her problems with Devon. The following exchange was recorded in my field notes.

> Devon, a 10-year-old boy, quietly worked on his project, a book about good things about starting school in the fall. His mother, Ms. Reed, sat beside him. Her lips were pursed, her eyes periodically darted around the room; there was a restlessness about her. She periodically made comments about her son's work that he interpreted as insulting. "Is that supposed to be a computer?" she said sarcastically. "That's not a nice thing to say to someone," Devon reprimanded. A little later, she commented, "That boy only has three fingers." Devon added more fingers in response. Ms. Reed tensely laughed and said, "Now, he has six fingers!" Devon face flushed; he looked down and said, "There are now five fingers on each hand. That is a mark on the paper, not a finger!"

After Devon finished drawing the pictures for his book, he asked his mother to help him punch holes in his paper because he wasn't able to squeeze the hole puncher with enough force to go through all the pages. After the holes were punched, Ms. Reed took the papers to lace them into a book as Devon was straightening up his work area. He looked over at her and tensed his face and said, "I want to lace it up a different way than you. Let me do it." Ms. Reed laughed tightly, rolled her eyes, and handed the book to Devon.

A CONVERSATION:
RESEARCH QUESTIONS, FINDINGS AND THE LITERATURE

After writing about caregiver distance in parent-child interactions described in the "Odd Child Out" subtheme, I went back to read professional literature to help me better understand what I observed. I re-examined the literature about the bi-directional nature of parent-child interaction that suggests that the caregivers may have been responding to a history of difficult interaction (Bugental, Caporeal, & Shennum, 1980; Greene & Doyle, 1999; Mash, 1984). Their expectations of interactions with their children may be that trouble will ensue if they have a reciprocal interaction. Cook, Kenny, and Goldstein (1991) reported in their study that adolescents elicited negative parental affect; it wasn't just that parents initiated the negative interaction. More intervention may need to occur with these families to help the children draw their caregivers toward them and to elicit positive caregiver affect to facilitate change in caregiver expectations.

Prior to this study, I believed that the manner in which parents and children interact in parent-child group might be a measure of how they interact with each other at home. After studying a few families in depth and after talking with some other parents, I no longer think that how parents and children interact in a structured parent-child group is a viable measure of typical parent-child interaction styles. Gardner's (2000) study supports this conclusion. She found that though the presence of an observer may not change the nature of the interactions, a structured or artificial setting for interactions elicits patterns that may not be representative of how parents and children interact at home. Both the parents and children reported that their experiences of interacting with each other in the parent-child group were different from their prior experiences of interacting with each other. This is due, in part, to the different cultures of the home and hospital environments.

Related to my emerging subquestion, "How do parents and children interact with each other in the parent-child activity group?," Mohr and Regan-Kubinski (2001) found that the parents of children with mental illness experienced chronic sorrow and demonstrated phases of grief that may be similar to what has been described about the behavior of the parents of children with severe physical or cognitive disabilities (Blacher, 1984; Featherstone, 1980; Wilker, Wasow, & Hatfield, 1981). They suggest that considering states of grieving may be another way of interpreting parents' behavior toward their children. For example, anger has been identified as one stage of the process of grieving. This study provoked my thinking about how the leaders of parent-child activity groups understand and interpret the parents' behavior, and how misinterpretation may lead to interventions that may inadvertently distance parents from leaders, or to no intervention at all. Parents sometimes interacted with their children in the parent-child activity group in a distant, frustrated, or angry manner. Considering the stages of grieving that parents may be experiencing may help the leaders of parent-child activity groups to reframe their views about angry interactions between a parent and child, and modify their approach to intervention.

Behavior that may initially be understood as demonstrating ineffective or dysfunctional caregiving may be viewed alternatively as a grief response. Though the goal of interventions related to helping parents find pleasure in their interactions with their children may remain the same, viewing parents' behavior as partially a grief response to their children's mental illness may strengthen the rapport between parents and group leaders. It may also encourage leaders to be more active and hopeful about the possibility of fostering change in a parent-child relationship.

During the course of my study, I read literature about emotional availability between parents and children. Many of my observations of parents and their children in interaction within the parent-child group fit into the categories that Biringen (2000) identify as "emotional availability." This concept is used to describe the degree of emotional openness and emotional communication between parent and child. Issues include the parents' sensitivity to their children, their ability to structure children's play, and the presence of expressions of hostility and intrusiveness toward their children. The children's behavior toward their parents is examined relative to children's involvement with their parents, their responsiveness to their parents, and the children's degree of hostility toward them.

I wrote about sensitive caregiving such as Teresa's approach to Joseph, as well as about incidents in which parents were less sensitive. Jason's mother Sally seemed to harbor a great deal of hostility toward her son. I found Betty, Tyrone's adoptive mother, to be insensitive toward Tyrone. She seemed intrusive to me as she criticized his work and demanded that he follow her lead. I also reported on the different ways that children were involved with their parents, and their responsiveness to their caregivers' requests and demands. For example, Sam was openly hostile to his mother, Pat, and was not involved in any activity with her. Pat expressed feeling frustration with Sam, and stated that she did not want to attend the parent-child group when Sam acted this way. Pat did not return to the parent-child group after a particularly difficult evening with Sam.

Changes in parent-child interaction reported by both parents and children may be framed as elements of emotional availability. Betty stated that she learned a great deal about Tyrone through interacting with him in the parent-child group. Both Betty and Tyrone felt that she was more open and involved with him at discharge than she was prior to his hospitalization because of their experiences in the parent-child group. They stated that they enjoyed their time together in the group. Tyrone worked hard in the parent-child group to listen to his adoptive mother's directions and engage in activity with her. In a future study, it may be productive to examine whether categorizing data collected in the parent-child activity group within the framework of emotional availability is helpful in analyzing data about parent-child interaction in a parent-child activity group and as a way to document change over time.

Over the course of my study, I also reflected on how the observations of parent-child interaction in the parent-child group and what participants reported about their interactions informed one another. I found that there were at times large differences between how leaders or I interpreted parent-child interaction within the group and what the parents and children reported. As I described in the last chapter, Rasheem's mother described one evening in parent-child group as a very positive experience for her family while Ruth reported the same family interactions as very troubled. At the beginning of Timmy's hospitalization, Mike and Timmy appeared to be enjoying their time together in parent-child group. However, Mike described his interactions with Timmy in parent-child group at this time as tense because he was always waiting for Timmy to have an outburst. In my logs, I described Betty's interactions with her adoptive son Tyrone as somewhat hostile, but both Tyrone and Betty reported that they enjoyed their time together in the parent-child group. Betty said that they had never spent time doing activities together before coming to the group. It is therefore important for leaders of a parent-child activity group to explore parent and child perceptions of their interactions within the group and how what they experience within the group resonates with their history of interaction prior to hospitalization. Interactions that appear negative to an observer may feel positive to parents and children whose experiences with each other have been harsher, colder, or more distant prior to hospitalization. Conversely, interactions that appear positive may in fact be stressful for a parent or child.

INFLUENCE OF MANAGED CARE

As I reflect upon what I reported about the leaders' interventions in this chapter, I feel that it is important to comment about how I experienced the impact of Managed Care on the participants of this study. Though a full discussion of the present issues in health care is beyond the scope of this chapter, how the changes in the mental health care system in the United States affected child psychiatric treatment at Green Hills and in turn how the parent-child activity group was led during my study, are important to mention. One clinician with whom I talked in passing, described present child inpatient psychiatric treatment as fast food treatment. When I mentioned this comment to Beth, she laughed and said that she agreed. Many of the children and parents that I observed had little time to adjust and make use of a therapy group like the parent-child group.

When I was a leader, children were typically hospitalized for at least two months and often stayed three or more months depending on placement issues. If children returned to the inpatient unit for a second time, there was usually a year or more between hospitalizations. In this study, four children were hospitalized two or more times over the course of my eight-month study. The necessary plans for the children's successful reintegration into their families were not completed at discharge. Once children were considered medically stable, they waited at home while school, camp, or therapy plans were finalized. At times, parents were so preoccupied about precipitous discharge plans that they could not focus on interacting with their children in the parent-child activity group.

When I was a leader of the parent-child activity group, I was encouraged by my supervisors to reflect upon my observations in the parent-child activity group so that I might provide interventions to the best of my ability. Group supervision was a routine part of every clinician's work experience. I was not supervised for the parent-child group, but I was supervised for other therapy groups that I led. I wrote process notes after many of the group sessions that I led and expected that the therapists that I, in turn, supervised did the same. After each parent-child activity group, I wrote logs about each family and shared my thoughts about the group process with my co-leader. Before each group, we met and discussed the families that might potentially attend the group that evening, chose a structured activity and considered which activities we might want to have available for the free play period of the group. The structure of Christine's job allowed her time for some reflection and interaction with children's therapists so that she too could think about ways that she might best help the families in the parent-child activity group.

Both Beth and Ruth described running from activity group to activity group. They did not describe any time in their daily schedules for reflection and did not expect such time. They stated how much they enjoyed sharing their experiences with me; it was a structured time that they reflected upon the parent-child group. Beth reported how she had taken time to plan for the group and discuss it afterwards when she co-led with Joan, her former supervisor. In our discussions, Beth described how she missed this experience. During this study, she did not plan each group with her co-leaders and did not discuss the group process with them after group sessions. She reported that she and her leaders were pressed for time. This was unfortunate for Ruth, Maria, a new social worker, and Sara and Martha, the occupational therapy students, because they were not trained to lead a parent-child activity group and were left to use their own academic and life experiences to guide their work. They did not have academic knowledge or supervised clinical experience about the issues of parents and their children with mental illness. Soo (1998) stated that without supervisory support, new therapists may not learn from their mistakes and may continue to repeat them. With limited success with their group interventions, untrained group leaders are likely to experience frustration and despair. A spontaneous comment that Maria made to me resonated with Soo's comment. She said, "I'm not sure what my role is here and if we even have an impact on these families."

What I have described about the barrier of Managed Care has been described elsewhere. Burns, Hoagwood, and Mrazek (1999) reviewed research suggesting that the shorter lengths of inpatient psychiatric stay since Managed Care has controlled mental health care resources limiting the effectiveness of services. This includes the actual length of time that patients are allowed to recover from a psychiatric crises and the time that professionals have to assess, develop and institute adequate plans to meet their patients' needs for support and intervention after hospitalization. The outcome is increased re-hospitalizations. Without having resolved the issues of an original psychiatric crisis that precipitated a psychiatric hospitalization, it is very likely that another crisis will soon occur. This was observed for some of the children in this study. In the process of multiple short term hospitalizations, both caregivers and children grew more distant from each other, and caregivers less hopeful about the possibility for positive change in their lives with their children.

REFERENCES

Blacher, J. (1984). Sequential stages of parental adjustment to the birth of a child with handicaps: Facts or artifact? *Mental Retardation, 22,* 55-68.

Bugental, D. B., Caporael, L., & Shennum, W. A. (1980). Experimentally produced child uncontrollability: Effects on the potency of adult communication patterns. *Child Development, 51,* 520-528.

Burns, B. J., Hoagwood, K., & Mrazek, P. J. (1999). Effective treatment for mental disorders in children and adolescents. *Clinical Child and Family Psychology Review, 2,* 199-254.

Cook, W. L., Kenny, D. A., & Goldstein, M. J. (1991). Parental affective style risk and the family system: A social relations model analysis. *Journal of Abnormal Psychology, 100,* 492-501.

Evans, S. (2001). Keeping safe: Supervision and support. In L. Lougher (Ed.). *Occupational therapy for child and adolescent mental health* (pp. 221-238). Edinburgh: Churchill Livingstone.

Featherstone, H. (1980). *A difference in the family: Life with a disabled child.* NY: Basic Books.

Gambrill, E. D. (1990). *Critical thinking in clinical practice: Improving the accuracy of judgments and decisions about clients.* San Francisco: Jossey-Bass.

Gardner, F. (2000). Methodological issues in the direct observation of parent-child interaction: Do observational findings reflect the natural behavior of participants? *Clinical Child and Family Psychology Review, 3,* 185-198.

Greene, R. W., & Doyle, A. E. (1999). Toward a transactional conceptualization of oppositional defiant disorder: Implications for assessment and treatment. *Clinical Child and Family Psychology Review, 2,* 129-148.

Mash, E. J. (1984). Families with problem children [Children in families under stress]. *New Directions for Child Development, 24,* 65-82.

Mohr, W. K., & Regan-Kubinski, M. J. (2001). Living in the fallout: Parents' experiences when their child becomes mentally ill. *Archives of Psychiatric Nursing, 15,* 69-77.

Soo, E. S. (1998). Is training and supervision of children and adolescents group therapists necessary? *Journal of Child and Adolescent Group Therapy, 8,* 181-196.

Wikler, L., Wasow, M., & Hatfield, E. (1981). Chronic sorrow revisited: Parent vs. professional depiction of the adjustment of parents of mentally retarded children. *American Journal of Orthopsychiatry, 51,* 63-70.

doi:10.1300/J004v22n03_06

Chapter 7

Parent-Child Activity Groups Reconsidered

SUMMARY. The influence of culture within a parent-child activity group is analyzed in order to explore how leaders of parent-child activity groups can use knowledge of group culture to design effective interventions. This chapter concludes with the author describing revisions to her original guidelines for parent-child activity group intervention which developed through her reflections on the findings of her qualitative study about one parent-child activity group. doi:10.1300/J004v22n03_07 *[Article copies available for a fee from The Haworth Document Delivery Service: 1-800-HAWORTH. E-mail address: <docdelivery@haworthpress.com> Website: <http://www.HaworthPress.com> © 2006 by The Haworth Press, Inc. All rights reserved.]*

KEYWORDS. Parent-child activity groups, therapeutic group culture, group leadership

ISSUES OF CULTURE

As I completed the analysis of the data of my qualitative study about one parent-child activity group, I searched for an overarching metatheme

---

[Haworth co-indexing entry note]: "Parent-Child Activity Groups Reconsidered." Olson, Laurette. Co-published simultaneously in *Occupational Therapy in Mental Health* (The Haworth Press, Inc.) Vol. 22, No. 3/4, 2006, pp. 103-119; and: *Activity Groups in Family-Centered Treatment: Psychiatric Occupational Therapy Approaches for Parents and Children* (Laurette Olson) The Haworth Press, Inc., 2006, pp. 103-119. Single or multiple copies of this article are available for a fee from The Haworth Document Delivery Service [1-800- HAWORTH, 9:00 a.m. - 5:00 p.m. (EST). E-mail address: docdelivery@haworthpress.com].

that would capture the essence of all of the themes that emerged about the experiences of the participants. The differences in the experiences between what parents reported happened at home and in parent-child activity group vividly stood out to me. I thought about culture–the home culture of families that include children with mental illness, the culture of the parent-child activity group and the institution in which it is embedded. In this chapter, I will describe how participating in a therapeutic group may be likened to a cultural voyage for persons who are new to a psychiatric institution based on the data collected in this study. My focus is how parents viewed and became acculturated to the group. The parent-child activity group was typically the parents' only opportunity to participate in a therapeutic group at Green Hills Hospital. On the other hand, their children participated in many groups and were immersed in the hospital culture. Viewing my data through the lens of culture opened up different possibilities to better understand the behavior of group members beyond the characteristics of parent-child interactional difficulties. Though my findings are specific to the participants of this study, other group leaders may find that my comments about institutional and group culture resonate with their own experiences of leading therapeutic groups at psychiatric institutions.

CULTURE DEFINED

A group's culture has been defined as including the values, language and experience that a group of people share and that differentiate them from other groups of people (Bonder, Martin, & Miracle, 2002). The values of a group have an impact upon how the members of the group view their experiences, interact with each other, and go about their daily activities. Members are insiders who readily interact with each other. Everyone else is considered an outsider and stranger. Outsiders may hold different values, have different languages or apply different meanings to common words, and may interpret experiences differently than the insiders do. They often interact uncomfortably or cautiously with insiders.

Though culture is considered as a factor in the provision of psychiatric services when clients and therapists have different ethnic or racial identities (Canino & Spurlock, 1994; Sue & Sue, 1990), it is also important to consider therapists as being insiders of the culture of psychiatric institutions and services, while clients may be outsiders. Mental health clinicians value the services they offer, speak the language of psychiatry, and have high status within the culture. Patients may not understand how services are intended to help them or the jargon used by clinicians about patients' mental illness. Patient status is lower than that of the mental health professionals who may be revered as experts who have the power to cure mental illness and help patients improve their daily lives. By participating in the therapeutic sessions offered by professionals, patients are initiated into the culture of the psychiatric hospital. They, then, become insiders, but their caregivers may remain outsiders to that culture.

Mental health clinicians participate in specific activities that are designed to identify mental illness and treat their patients. Leading a therapeutic group is one such activity. Groups provide an organized way for clinicians to assess patients' interaction with other people and then help patients improve their interaction skills. How the group leaders direct conversation and the activities that they provide for group members suggest what they value and by extension, what is valued within the group. Over time, these groups develop a culture of their own.

THE CULTURE OF THE PARENT-CHILD ACTIVITY GROUP

A central value of the parent-child activity group is that positive parent-child interaction in everyday activities is critical to children's mental health. If positive parent-child interaction occurs frequently, children are more apt to exhibit a positive mood, be compliant with directions from caregivers, and be interested in play and activity. The assumption is that many parents and children have not been able to enjoy pleasurable joint leisure activities prior to hospitalization. This assumption guides what occurs in the group. Parents and children are offered activities in which they can experience mutual pleasurable benign interaction. Within the group, parents and children are expected to work collaboratively, engage in social conversations while they participate in activities, clean up their workspaces at the end of activities, and be amenable to the direction and guidance of the leaders.

Norms of behavior within the parent-child activity group are different from the behavior parents reported about their parent-child interaction at home. In the group, completing a task with their children and playing a game with them are expected parental behaviors. Prior to the hospitalization, participation in such activities was not expected. Parents, such as Mike, Andrea, and Kathy, described their focus on managing their children's disruptive, resistive behavior. Mike and Carlos' father described themselves as hostages to their children's behavior. They stayed home to avoid being embarrassed in public, avoided their children when they were quiet and spent a great deal of time reprimanding them. What they considered acceptable behavior at home changed as their children's mental illness worsened. They expected little of their children. Kathy and Mike, for example, reported bathing their school age children.

Some parents and children found the structured environment of the parent-child group welcome and enjoyed the different behavioral expectations. Participating in the group felt good to them. They were expected to approach each other positively and engage in benign conversation. This opened a door to interacting with each other that was different from what they had grown accustomed to at home. They shared or developed values that the parent-child activity group was designed to reinforce; they accepted the behavioral norms of the group. Mike thought that it was important for parents to play with their children, but acknowledged that prior to Timmy's hospitalization, he rarely played with his son. At the beginning of Timmy's hospitalization, Mike could not relax or play with Timmy because he expected his son to have a temper tantrum at any moment. Mike persevered. Over time, participating with his son in the group became an enjoyable time with his son. He regularly shared his feelings about interacting with Timmy with me. As he reflected upon their interactions, he may have reconsidered his expectations as Timmy's symptoms of mental illness receded. He began to look for new ways to interact with Timmy productively. Not all parents became comfortable participating with their children in the parent-child activity group; the group culture may have felt strange to them. These individuals attended only one or two groups and had little interaction with their children during the group. Some brought other children to the group with whom they interacted more easily.

CONSIDERING VANTAGE

In examining any group of people, it is important to consider vantage. Vantage is each person's unique perspective on an experience (Bonder, Martin, & Miracle, 2002). Each person's point of view is based not only on his or her own values and assumptions, but also upon their position within or outside the culture, as well as on the individual's particular focus at that time. Even parents who became insiders and accepted the values of the parent-child activity group, perceived what occurred in the group quite differently than the leaders did. Parents have a lower status than leaders in the overall culture of the Green Hills Hospital and the leaders have the power to affect how other insiders, including the children's psychiatrists, view parents and children. For these reasons, parents may be hesitant to question leaders' behavior. They may not agree with leaders' approaches to managing children or their choices of group activities. When leaders do not work to understand the vantage of parents, they may develop an inaccurate view about what parents find acceptable or helpful. Silence may be mistaken as agreement with the leaders' point of view.

Leaders focus on their own ideal of parent-child activity interaction. During my research, I was struck by examples of the different foci of parents from that of the leaders. In some cases, when the leaders or I saw problems in interaction, parents reported improved interaction with their children. In Chapter 5, I compared what Rasheem's and Tyrone's mothers reported to me about their interactions with their sons and Ruth's and my perceptions of the same interactions. Unless leaders ask parents about their focus, they may intervene when parents may need support to provide support for their children. The leaders' feedback may result in decreased parent-child interaction because parents may perceive that what they were doing did not meet the leaders' standards for parent-child interaction and shut down what may have been a productive change in parent-child interaction from the parents' and children's perspectives. If this happens, the group then may lose some of its power to move parents and children toward more productive ways of interacting.

Because the parent-child activity group is embedded within a medical hospital, some of the caregivers' focus is evaluating whether medication has an effect. When parents focused primarily on observing the children's behavior for medication related changes, their interactions with the children are influenced by that expectation. They may be impatient or tense as they look for change related to medication effect as opposed to working toward changes in interaction related to ways of participation in activity with each other. Teresa's behavior toward her grandson Joseph, and her comments about him at the end of Joseph's second hospitalization during this study demonstrated this. The leaders need to be aware of the different focus of parent participants. They can use their knowledge to ease parents' concerns–empathize as well as work to alter what parents attend to in their interactions with their children.

WHEN CULTURAL DIFFERENCES ARE UNRECOGNIZED

Unrecognized differences in values, language, and experience can undermine productive interaction because persons from one culture may interpret the behaviors of another within the framework of their own culture. Group leaders may not recognize the ways in which group members' life experiences can alter values and expectations of behavior. They may expect that new group members will acclimate quickly to the group culture since they assume that group values are universally accepted. When members resist participation, leaders may interpret this as a symptom of mental illness or unwillingness to change.

Like Fadiman (1997) reported, professionals often feel that by the nature of their education and experience that they understand what is best for children. Parents are expected to comply with the guidelines of the treatment designed by professionals. Though parents may desire help in reducing their children's symptoms of mental illness, they may not agree that their way of interacting with their children need to change. Playing with their children may feel superfluous. When clinicians don't ask them directly about their views and expect them to participate in group treatment activities that they may not value or understand, treatment services may feel like coercion. An unbridgeable gap may be created between parents and the service providers. It may be more productive to think about parents who attend parent-child group with their children as visitors to a different culture that may sharply contrast with their previous life experience. This viewpoint may help to prompt clinicians to search for differences by observing carefully and talking directly to those for whom they provide services. Often, the similarities that clients share with professionals such as language, clothes, and country blur the professionals' ability to see other differences that may exist in values and experience.

GUIDES FOR THE VOYAGE

If the experience of parents and children in the parent-child activity group can be metaphorically considered a cultural voyage, then group leaders might optimally view themselves as cultural guides. Like any visitors who only have a short time to spend in a different culture, these group participants may need guides to help them become oriented to and appreciate the new culture.

First, guides must understand the strangers who have come to visit their culture. As insiders who welcome outsiders, guides must empathize with the discomfort or disorientation that visitors feel as they enter a different culture. What they see, may be dramatically different from their prior experiences and may even challenge their familiar way of interacting. To help the visitors feel comfortable, guides find ways to include visitors in the activities of the insiders of the culture. Guides explain how parents and children interact in the parent-child activity group and help the visitors find parallels in their own culture in spite of differences. In this way, guides help families make what feels unfamiliar, familiar. As guides watch the visiting parents and children participate in activities, they observe what draws the attention of the visitors and makes sense to them. Guides can then make educated guesses about what activities the visitors might enjoy experiencing during subsequent visits and that might help them make a connection to this new culture.

After listening carefully to how parents and children speak to each other and asking them questions when they don't understand, guides may become knowledgeable about the language that parents and children use among themselves. The guides can then facilitate conversation with parents and children about the similarities and differences that they observe between their typical ways of interacting and the ways that parents and children are encouraged to interact within the group. As the visitors see the guides working hard to understand their family culture, visitors can relax and be open to learning about the culture of the parent-child activity group. Over time, they may find the feelings experienced while participating in the activities of this culture so positive that they search for ways to bring what they learned back home. Those visitors whose stay within the culture of the parent-child group is very brief, may need further opportunities to visit a similar group after children's hospitalization before what they observed and experienced within the parent-child group becomes meaningful to them.

DISCUSSION

Parents who participated in this study reported large differences in their and their children's behavior in the group versus at home. Children appeared to be on their best behavior; the parents didn't yell as much. It is important that leaders be very cognizant of these disparities in experience. If leaders apply the metaphor of a cultural voyage, they may be more attentive to learning about the parents' and children's perspectives and be more conscious of the possibility that the parents and children view the experiences differently than the leaders. Through open discussion, parents may reflect upon what the differences in their children's and their own behavior might mean and how they might build upon any positive changes for improved positive interaction outside of the group. Without discussion, some parents may write off any positive differences that they observe in their children's behavior in the parent-child group as the child hiding their true behavior in the presence of the leaders.

Therapeutic groups are not frequently analyzed as separate cultures where the dynamics of culture affect the interactive process between clinicians and the recipients of service. The dynamics present in groups are most often related to the symptoms of mental illness that brought the recipients to the group and institution. The data from this study suggest that some of the discomfort, resistance, or withdrawal that leaders observed in parent participants' behavior may have been related to sharp differences in the cultural environment of the group relative to their home environment. Other leaders of therapeutic groups may find some similarities in my data to their experiences and may want to consider how the culture of their groups affects the behavior of their group participants. Guiding group participants through the process of acculturation to the group may open the door for participants to use more fully the services that group leaders offer.

Studies in the future might directly examine the culture of therapeutic groups such as a parent-child activity group. There is much to be learned about how recipients of mental health service are acculturated into these groups. More closely examining the vantage of professionals and the other group participants than I have been able might help group leaders provide services that are more welcoming to new members and increase their therapeutic value to recipients. This is especially true in the Managed Care climate where time constraints are placed on the participation of families in the mental health care system. Patients and their families may attend only a few groups and therefore their opportunity to acclimate to the groups and benefit from it is limited. Leaders need to be very cognizant of the viewpoints of group participants so that they can guide them in making a connection to the group and possibly finding something within it to apply to their life when they leave the institution.

RECONSIDERATION OF GUIDELINES
FOR A PARENT-CHILD ACTIVITY GROUP

Given the findings of this study, some parts of the original guidelines for practice are clearer to me as I consider them within the context of my data. The findings of the study emphasized to me the importance of carefully choosing activities and leaders' facilitating conversation. Prior to this study, I had not sufficiently reflected upon the environment of the group and how parents' and children's behavior may be very different with each other than it is at other times. Mohr's and Regan-Kubinski's 2001 study about the issues of grieving and constant sorrow in parents of children with mental illness has also changed how I think about the ways parents interact with their children in a parent-child activity group. Leaders of a parent-child activity group in a psychiatric facility need to reflect upon these issues as they think about how to help these parents interact with their children.

Some recommendations for refining parent-child group guidelines grew from the metathemes discussed in Chapters 5 and 6. The examples and discussion of my metathemes, "A door is opening" and "There are barriers blocking the door" led me to think about the importance of maximizing and capitalizing on the inherent elements of the group, including a different environment, children on their best behavior, the power of activity to change moods, and the presence of other families and the leaders for support and observations, as well as how leaders might facilitate family interaction. As I wrote about my overarching metatheme, "Therapeutic groups are cultural voyages," which I discussed earlier in this chapter, I became convinced that, above all, it is critical for leaders to explore their own culture as clinicians and employees of a psychiatric institution and to consider how disconcerting it may be for families to enter this culture. With a greater awareness of cultural differences, therapists will likely pursue knowledge about parents' values and experiences with children. Then they will be in a position to help parents and children understand the values of the parent-child activity group and to use the parent-child activity group in their own ways to experience positive and productive interactions with each other.

THE ENVIRONMENT

A different but structured and safe environment seemed to provoke changes in how some parents and children interacted with each other.

The changes often were positive. Both parents and children often commented on this.

A parent-child activity group might, therefore, provide the opportunity to make some inroads into breaking the negative cycle of interaction to which the literature refers relative to children with behavioral disorders and their parents. It may be important to acknowledge the difference in a child's behavior in the presence of their parents, especially in the case of parents who believe that the child's positive changes are just a ruse. Greater responsiveness and willingness to engage with their parents in a structured environment does not negate the presence of serious behavioral problems that children exhibited prior to hospitalization, and may continue to exhibit after discharge from the hospital. More emotional availability on the part of the child in the parent-child group may open a door for better communication between them, which in turn may lead to a better opportunity for parents to influence their children's behavior.

Parents may be more open in relating to their children in the parent-child group, because they are less stressed by the multiple demands of home or the presence of other children. Parents may also feel nurtured by the leaders who provide activity and a structure through which they can interact with their children. In the process, a leader might also gently help a parent see how they too might be behaving differently because of the environment of the group and come to see how their behavior and mood affects their children. Borrego and Urquiza (1998) suggest that the leaders may provide social reinforcement for parents from a behavioral point of view. This may mediate change in how the parents interact with their children. With the support, guidance, and reinforcement from the leaders and other parents in the process of interacting with their children through play and activity, parents may begin to interact with their children differently and see the importance of spending time with their children in this way.

The presence of additional family members in addition to a parent and child changes the social environment of the group. The leaders may need to change how family members sit in relation to each other and how the group activity is structured. During the course of my study, I found observing hospitalized children with their caregivers who brought other children in the family to the parent-child activity group particularly poignant. In Chapter 6, I described how some caregivers sat next to and focused on non-hospitalized children within the group, leaving the hospitalized children to work independently. As described in the literature (Preston, 1990), parents may not expect to have positive interactions with their children with mental illness and may have the opportunity to avoid interactions with these children when other children are present. It is important that leaders help parents and children have the opportunity to interact by first carefully seating family members so that interaction between hospitalized children and their primary caregivers is probable, and then by choosing activities that will foster conversation and interaction.

THE ACTIVITIES

Activities must be skillfully chosen and used by leaders in order to engage parents with their children. Many families that include a child with mental illness have experienced failure in their attempts to participate in mutual activity (Olson, 1999, 2001). A novel, interesting activity that requires some new learning, but is not overly challenging, has been observed to lead to greater interaction between parents and children. In some cases, the mood of some angry parents and children lightened, allowing increased interaction in play to occur. When the leaders resorted to using easy, ready-made projects that just required coloring, parents and children remained sullen and involved with each other. In the gym, the leaders infrequently offered different activities instead of things like basketball, which was regularly played by the children. When they introduced novel activities that were within the capacity of the family members, more positive responses were elicited. Ruth noted, "Sometimes basketball just doesn't do it for families."

In Chapter 6, I described a range of ways that the choice of activities appeared to be an interactional barrier between parents and children. The choice of activity requires consideration of not only what interests and is developmentally appropriate for particular children, but also what will foster the engagement of children with their parents. Open-ended projects are attractive to children because children choose the theme of their projects and decide how the projects will look. Some element of choice is particularly important for children with psychiatric disorders since many children who are hospitalized exhibit oppositional or resistant behavior to demands from adults. Open-ended projects often promote children to seek adult help in organizing and planning the task. Close-ended projects do not; the task requirements are explicit. Rasheem refused to participate one night when the activity involved coloring dinosaur puzzles because he did not like dinosaurs. When he was allowed to design his own puzzle, he was willing to participate in the activity and sought out the help of his mother and sister. Turning a close-ended activity into one that allowed him some power to design his own project fostered Rasheem's engagement in activity and through the activity, with his mother and sister. Gary was certainly interested in painting a wooden car, but the task was a solitary one that left Gary and his mother unengaged with each other.

Parents' role in activities is also an important consideration. The activities chosen must also be ones for which parents have the capacity and interest to participate. Leaders must find ways to help parents when parents require assistance in completing an activity without taking over the parental role. Parents may need help to redirect children to a different activity due to either the parents' or the children's needs for organized or quiet activity.

The use of play and activity in a parent-child activity group requires a complex understanding of the uses of play and activity for building skills in children and also for fostering interactions between parents and children. Due to the deficits that some of the children exhibit relative to impulsivity, short attention span, low frustration tolerance, and limited skill development, leaders must also be skilled in assisting parents to modify activities.

FACILITATING CONVERSATION

The presence of other families can be a potential asset to helping families interact and to open new doors for parents and children. When parents identified with the conversations or interactions of other parents with their children or a leader, it seemed to have a powerful effect. Leaders need to take an active role in facilitating conversation, and guiding and shaping the direction of the conversations. There were a few examples of this in my study, especially when Christine was a co-leader of the group. One example of this occurred when Mr. Boland listened as Christine talked with Jenny and her family about sibling rivalry and provocation between siblings. The conversation resonated with Mr. Boland's experiences with his own children. He joined the conversation and reflected with other members about his new ways of thinking about what happens among siblings and how to manage these interactions within a family. Tom smiled and listened quietly as his father talked with the leaders and other parents.

In thinking about conversation in the group, the leaders should consider how conversation reflects culture: the cultures of children who are psychiatrically hospitalized and parents who have children who are psychiatrically hospitalized, as well as the cultures of families and the leaders. This is an opportunity for leaders to learn about the different cultures with which the parents and children identify as well as to reflect upon how their own culture as leaders and staff members of Green Hills impacts on their opinions and interactions with group participants. Leaders then have increased knowledge to use for building a collaborative relationship with parents and children in the interest of developing a parent-child activity group culture that opens doors for positive interaction between parents and children.

The analogy of prison that Rasheem, Joseph, and Gary used to describe their experience of being psychiatrically hospitalized is the same analogy used by persons who were psychiatrically hospitalized as children when they described their experiences to another researcher (Mohr, 1999). This conversation may have provided the leaders, as well as the parents with an opportunity to better understand how children experience psychiatric hospitalization and to learn more about the subculture experienced by the children. By pursuing the conversation, the adults might have helped the children better understand the reasons for their hospitalization, as well as providing an opportunity for the children to express their anger about being "locked up." A conversation like this might have also helped the parents to develop ways to talk more openly with their children about their concerns.

Conversation should be facilitated within families as well as across families when appropriate. Conversation occurs spontaneously as parents and children work together on an activity, and the opportunity to simultaneously observe other families working on similar activities promotes conversation as well. Parents and children may also identify with the comments that they overhear between other parents and children. Leaders need to be prepared to participate in spontaneous conversation as appropriate and guide conversation toward helping parents and children elaborate on topics important to the children, finding similarities in experiences among families and helping to guide the resolution of task or interpersonal conflicts as necessary.

CONSIDERING ISSUES OF PARENTS' CONSTANT SORROW

My data related to what parents reported about their interactions with their psychiatrically hospitalized children are consonant with what Mohr and Regan-Kubinski (2001) suggested may be related to chronic sorrow or the process of grieving. Leaders of a parent-child activity group should be aware that these parents may be going through stages of grief similar to the experiences of parents of children with physical disabilities. In the initial stages of grief, parents of children with physical disabilities may exhibit less pleasure in parenting, tendencies to reject offspring with disabilities, and lowered confidence in caring for children with disabilities. Some of the same behaviors observed in the parents of children with mental illness may also be reflective of these initial stages of grief.

If leaders can identify the stage of grief and then match their interventions to helping a parent work through that stage, then the parents may be better able to experience positive feelings, to see the positive features that remain in their children, and begin to enjoy parent-child interaction. Drotar, Baskiewicz, Irvin, Kennell, and Klaus (1975) pointed out that there is ambivalence in each stage of grief. Feelings may vacillate between despair and hope, rejection and attachment, or anger and equanimity. For example, this is evident in Kathy's description of her feelings and actions toward her son, Ian, which was described in Chapter 5. More research specifically related to how grief may impact the interactions between parents and children with mental illness is needed.

THOUGHTS ABOUT THE EDUCATION OF LEADERS

Leaders learned how to lead the group by doing, and were not observed to reflect on their experiences with each other. At the end of the group, leaders straightened up the group room, escorted families back to the unit, wrote notes, and reported to nursing staff about any incidences that occurred in group that might affect the children's behavior on the unit. They did not have discussions among themselves about what went well in the group and what they might do differently next time to better help the parents and children interact with each other. Leaders were typically willing to sit down after group with me and discuss their thoughts about the evening, but I did not observe them doing the same with each other. Leaders seemed to enjoy the process of reflecting upon their observations of parents and children after group sessions. It is possible that our discussions were helpful as they worked with families over time.

A post-group discussion is considered a necessity by group therapy experts, especially when leaders have one year or less of experience with a group (Yalom, 1995). When thinking about the parent-child activity group, all of the therapists but Beth had less than one year of experience with the group. In Yalom's study of 12 nonprofessionally trained group leaders in a psychiatric hospital, half of the leaders received on-going supervision and training and the other half simply led their groups. Besides finding that the trained therapists demonstrated improved skill at the end of six months, he found that the therapists who did not receive any training were less skilled at the end of the six months. His conclusion was that simple experience is not enough to develop competency in leading a therapeutic group. Without supervision, "original errors may be reinforced by simple repetition" (Yalom, 1995, p. 516). This study resonates with my experience. When a clinical supervisor is not available to help leaders reflect upon the therapeutic group experience they provide, discussing and critically analyzing what occurs in group sessions with co-leaders enhance group leaders' skill development.

When I initiated the parent-child activity group, there were no clinicians available to supervise my co-leader and myself around our group practice. Instead, we reflected upon the parent-child activity group through group notes and post-group discussions weekly. We reviewed our group notes periodically so that we could better understand the process that we perceived families experienced from week to week. During the course of this research, Beth said that she felt that her leadership of the parent-child activity group was most effective when she co-led the group with her former supervisor, Joan. Beth described how they discussed families and what occurred in the group and made plans for subsequent groups based upon these discussions.

In my experience, when an individual leads a group routinely without reflection, it is likely that he or she will miss the richness of the interactions that occur within the group and overlook opportunities to influence those interactions. As Yalom (1995) demonstrated, poor leadership habits can develop without the leader's awareness. I saw this occurring with the leadership of the parent-child activity group over the length of my study. After Christine left and new leaders began to assist Beth, at times a secondary group developed during the parent-child group. Sometimes, leaders would stand away from the group table and talk about miscellaneous topics between themselves while the families were working on their projects. A few times, a leader or a student tried to draw me into their conversation. Near the end of my study, the two primary leaders decided that they would wrap Christmas presents for the children and leave Maria, a brand new leader, to run the parent-child group alone. At times, the role of the leaders was reduced to providing materials and supervising families to ensure their safety, rather than interacting with the families to promote positive interaction. This behavior contrasted with what they reported about their beliefs related to the function of the parent-child activity group.

I strongly believe that anyone planning to lead a parent-child activity group should also plan how they will develop their leadership skills for the group. It is critical to have academic and clinical training in working with children as well as in group process and in the therapeutic use of play.

As an occupational therapist, I wrote the initial guidelines for practice in a way that used the strengths of my academic and clinical background. Education in occupational therapy includes in-depth study about the occupations of persons across the lifespan and how to use activities to promote the occupational functioning of persons with physical or psychiatric disability or at risk for developing disability.

Occupational therapists learn to modify activities and the environment so that persons with disabilities can participate in everyday living along with other people in their families and communities. With this type of education, a group leader is sensitive to facets of the environment and activity that may support or promote function, as well as the facets that may inhibit function when a person has a disability. As a leader of a parent-child activity group, an occupational therapist may be more likely to recognize the need to modify an activity or the group environment so that children can participate in the activity with their parents. Analyzing the environment or activity in depth so that the needs of an adult to successfully parent a child with mental illness is an elaboration of thinking that occupational therapists are trained to do.

REFERENCES

Bonder, B., Martine, L., & Miracle, A. (2002). *Culture in Clinical Care*. Thorofare, NJ: Slack.

Borrego, J., & Urquiza, A. J. (1998). Importance of therapist use of social reinforcement with parents as a model for parent-child relationships: An example with parent-child interaction therapy. *Child & Family Behavior Therapy, 20(4)*, 27-54.

Canino, I. A. & Spurlock, J. (1994). *Culturally Diverse Children and Adolescents: Assessment, Diagnosis, and Treatment*. NY: Guilford Press.

Drotar, P., Baskiewicz, A., Irvin, N., Kennell, J., & Klaus, M. (1975). The adaptation of parents to the birth of an infant with a congenital malformation: A hypothetical model. *Pediatrics, 56*, 710-717.

Fadiman, A. (1997). *The spirit catches you and you fall down*. NY: Farrar, Straus, & Giroux.

Mohr, W. K. (1999). Discovering a dialectic of care, *Western Journal of Nursing Research, 21,* 225-245.

Mohr, W. K., & Regan-Kubinski, M. J. (2001). Living in the fallout: Parents' experiences when their child becomes mentally ill. *Archives of Psychiatric Nursing, 15,* 69-77.

Olson, L. (1999). Psychosocial frame of reference. In P. Kramer & J. Hinojosa (Eds.), *Frames of reference for pediatric occupational therapy* (2nd Ed., pp. 323-375). Baltimore, MD: Williams and Wilkins.

Olson, L. (2001). Child psychiatry in the USA. In L. Lougher (Ed.), *Occupational Therapy for Child and Adolescent Mental Health* (pp. 173-191). Edinburgh: Churchill Livingstone.

Preston, T. (1990). Parents' perceptions of behavior in disturbed children: A study of attributions, affect, and expectancies. (Doctoral dissertation, Vanderbilt University, 1990). *Dissertation Abstracts International, 51,* (5-B) 2632.

Sue, D. W. & Sue, D. (1990). *Counseling the Culturally Different: Theory and Practice* (2nd Ed.). NY: John Wiley & Sons.

Yalom, I. D. (1995). *The Theory and Practice of Group Psychotherapy* (4th Ed.). NY: Basic Books.

doi:10.1300/J004v22n03_07

Chapter 8

Engaging Psychiatrically Hospitalized Teens with Their Parents Through a Parent-Adolescent Activity Group

SUMMARY. What the literature reports that adolescents need within their parent-adolescent relationships, as well as what adolescents with serious emotional disturbances may experience within their parent-adolescent relationships are discussed. A framework for providing parent-adolescent group intervention for psychiatrically hospitalized adolescents and their parents to promote positive interaction and co-occupation are provided. Summaries of the parent-adolescent activity group experiences of three families are provided to illustrate how different adolescent psychiatric issues and family dynamics might be addressed in a parent adolescent activity group. doi:10.1300/J004v22n03_08 *[Article copies available for a fee from The Haworth Document Delivery Service: 1-800-HAWORTH. E-mail address: <docdelivery@haworthpress.com> Website: <http://www.HaworthPress.com> © 2006 by The Haworth Press, Inc. All rights reserved.]*

KEYWORDS. Inpatient adolescent psychiatric treatment, parent-adolescent interaction, occupational therapy

---

[Haworth co-indexing entry note]: "Engaging Psychiatrically Hospitalized Teens with Their Parents Through a Parent-Adolescent Activity Group." Olson, Laurette. Co-published simultaneously in *Occupational Therapy in Mental Health* (The Haworth Press, Inc.) Vol. 22, No. 3/4, 2006, pp. 121-133; and: *Activity Groups in Family-Centered Treatment: Psychiatric Occupational Therapy Approaches for Parents and Children* (Laurette Olson) The Haworth Press, Inc., 2006, pp. 121-133. Single or multiple copies of this article are available for a fee from The Haworth Document Delivery Service [1-800- HAWORTH, 9:00 a.m. - 5:00 p.m. (EST). E-mail address: docdelivery@haworthpress.com].

From birth and throughout childhood, the parent-child relationship is central to children's development of all adaptive skills. In combination with temperament and biological makeup, this first attachment relationship has correlated with children's and adolescent's development of coping skills, capacities for emotional regulation, peer competence (Sroufe, Carlson, & Shulman, 1993; Allen & Land, 1999) and more harmonious sibling relationships (Teti & Ablard, 1989). A study by Pettit, Bates, and Dodge (1997) suggested that supportive parenting (mother-to-child warmth, proactive teaching, inductive discipline and positive involvement) correlated with children's positive school adjustment and may buffer children from the negative effects of family adversity.

As children enter adolescence and begin to separate their identity from their families, tense parent-child relationships are expected and are often accepted as the status quo. Though more conflict is probable, stable and supportive interactions between parents and offspring are more often the norm. Adolescents gain a firm sense of identity and independence through a positive relationship with their parents.

Grotevant and Cooper (1985) stated that in contrast to traditional conceptualizations of breaking the parent-child bond, studies support the view of adolescence as a period of gradual renegotiation between parent and child from the asymmetrical authority of early and middle childhood toward a potentially peer-like mutuality in adulthood. Adolescent maturity is gained in the context of progressive and mutual redefinition of the parent-child relationship rather than by the adolescent simply leaving the relationship. Gullotta, Adams, and Markstrom (1999) reported that researchers have found that competent adolescents tend to have warm relations with their parents who are able to appropriately monitor and set limits with their behavior.

Communication, good family problem solving skills, and the ability to rework family relationships to accommodate the developmental changes and increasing competency in the adolescent are vital to parent-adolescent relationships that support adolescents' successful transition to adulthood. Landel (1990) stated that a warm, interactive and partially restricting family structure is best for healthy adolescent development. A study by Allen et al. (2003) suggested that an adolescent is most likely to be secure and able to explore autonomous functioning when the adolescents can discuss disagreements and their viewpoints within a supportive mother-child relationship. Allen, Hauser, Bell, and O'Connor (1994) suggest that for parents to facilitate their adolescent offspring's autonomous functioning, it is important that parents support their offspring's exploration of their different points of view as opposed to demanding conformity.

Adolescents in trouble often live in families that are not able to practice these behaviors. These families have frequent conflicts and tend to exhibit poor problem solving skills as a family. Their communication is typically defensive rather than supportive. In these families, conflict is stopped through withdrawal and silence rather than resolution (Montemayor, 1986). After reviewing the literature and considering their own research on adolescence, Gullotta, Adams, and Markstrom (1999) recommend that intervention programs for adolescents and their families emphasize and help families build cohesion, adaptiveness and communication into their family structure in order to optimally support adolescents' successful transition to adulthood. Zabriskie and McCormick's 2003 study suggested that family leisure activities may promote greater satisfaction with family life and may also support increased positive communication.

In a review of the critical issues facing the treatment of adolescents with serious emotional disturbances in residential facilities, Leichtman and Leichtman (2001) conclude that in order for these youths to develop the skills and relationships necessary for transitioning back to their families and communities, their families must be a central part of the treatment provided at the facilities. Cafferty and Leichtman (2001) suggest that the work of the team in residential care of adolescents needs to help youths focus on their goal of transitioning back to their communities or families throughout treatment and to serve a supporting role to families. They state that all members of the team should be prepared to work with families. Occupational therapists with their focus on promoting occupational participation should be active team members in helping families re-integrate their offspring with emotional disorders back into everyday family living.

A FRAMEWORK FOR PARENT-ADOLESCENT OCCUPATION-BASED GROUP INTERVENTION

A parent-adolescent occupation-based group was conceptualized to promote positive mutual relationships between parents and their hospitalized adolescents. It was developed from a similar group that was used with younger children and their families previously described in this book. This group was developed when young adolescents were hospitalized on the child inpatient unit, and their different needs for engaging with their parents were identified. These adolescents resisted the parent-child activity group stating that the idea was "stupid" and that they couldn't stand to do things with their parents. At the same time, they admitted that in order to return home, they needed to get along with their parents to some degree. An altered format for interactions with their parents within an activity group was negotiated.

The psychiatrically hospitalized adolescents interviewed for potentially participating in the parent-adolescent group reported feeling disconnected, criticized, infantilized, ignored, not supported, or intruded upon by their parents. Most reported not engaging in any satisfying mutual activity with either parent since they were young children. Some of their parents stated that they felt disconnected from their adolescent children and did not know how to positively engage or reach them through activity. Others reported feeling overwhelmed by the dependency of their child. Some denied having any problems interacting or doing activities with their offspring, while also describing a tense and unsatisfying relationship.

A parent-adolescent activity group is a multifamily group that may meet one time per week. Adolescents engage in a self-chosen activity with their parents parallel to other adolescents and their parents. The activity may be one that the adolescent enjoys, may be one that he or she may want to explore, or may be one they remember enjoying participating in with their parents and think that they still may enjoy. Parents are encouraged to support their adolescents' interests and exploration and to use the opportunity to learn more about what their adolescent was interested in and to use the experience of shared activity to promote a relaxed conversation.

Though families work parallel to one another, the elements of group process are very important to the functioning of the group. Families are generally supportive of each other since they are all "in the same boat." Within the group, families can observe the positive and negative interactions between other parent-adolescent dyads. This can be the most powerful intervention. A new family will model after a family that has been working within the group for a few weeks.

Meeting, observing, talking and working side by side with other families who have had similar experiences with a troubled adolescent, and have experienced positive change in their interactions during the adolescent's hospitalization instills hope. Observing negative interactions in other families can sensitize a parent or an adolescent to their own behavior. An adolescent may note that another adolescent is giving his parent a "hard" time and may empathize with that parent. At the same time that group members are observing other families, they are interacting with their own family members.

Though at times negative contagion does occur, the reflections on the immediate behavioral interactions of others in the here and now can lead to more positive behavior in the observer. When negative behavior of one adolescent with his parent encourages another adolescent to act similarly with his own parent, it is generally related to an adolescent developmental concern not being addressed within the group. An example of this is when a parent is openly critical and not listening to the verbal or nonverbal requests of an adolescent for more autonomy in the activity. If a leader does not facilitate a more positive and balanced interchange and that adolescent chooses to respond in a reciprocally negative manner to his parent's manner, other adolescents may join in and band against the perceived injustices of adults in general. These other adolescents may also choose the time to bring up similar complaints about their parents' behaviors leading to increasing the negative activity interactions between parents and adolescents. This dynamic is most evident when there are adolescents with conduct disorders within the group.

The elements of classical activity group therapy as defined by Slavson and Schiffer (1975) are also evident in this intervention approach. Activity group therapy is an experiential approach that provides the group membership with the opportunity for meaningful interpersonal activity-based interaction. Activity is the medium through which maladaptive behavior is modified and group members learn about ways to positively engage one another. Through the activity and the leaders' structure, support, and intervention around it, negative interaction styles are shaped to be more benign and positive. The possibility of change that may not have been considered before may now seem a possibility. Within the activity, family deficits in interacting become evident, but also strengths that may not have been noted may also become evident. The activity process may encourage family members to seek solutions to interactional difficulties around a concrete activity. With success with activity participation, satisfaction and pleasure in the accomplishment are shared by parent and adolescent.

ROLE OF THE LEADERS

The leaders:

1. Assist parent-adolescent dyads to choose, plan and initiate the implementation of a benign and potentially mutually pleasurable activity.
2. Remain accessible, but allow family members to figure out how to participate in the activity together.
3. Intervene and help a family organize and carry out the steps of an activity together if a family becomes stuck in a constraining interaction.
4. Facilitate conversation between parents and adolescents and if appropriate between different families.
5. Model respect for the rights and individuality of all group members.
6. Model and teach active listening and problem solving skills.
7. Increase parents' and adolescents' awareness of the verbal and nonverbal cues of each other.
8. Focus members on their roles as parents or adolescent offspring, and gently help shift the balance when roles become unbalanced or reversed.

The group leaders help parents prepare for the parent-adolescent activity group by providing a discussion group about what will occur and strategies for engaging their offspring and managing possible difficulties that may arise in their interactions with their children. Some expect resistance or rejection from their children. Changing their expectations so that they are more relaxed and open to their children is critical if negative cycles of parent-adolescent interaction are to be broken. Events of the last group session are also discussed to promote learning through reflection and reframe any negative feelings that may hinder interactions within the group. Parents set goals for interacting with their adolescent child for the evening.

CASE DESCRIPTIONS OF PARTICIPANTS OF THE PARENT-ADOLESCENT GROUP

Steve: Activity as a Bridge to Rebuild a Relationship

This was the first psychiatric admission for Steve, a 16-year-old boy who withdrew from all academic and social contact for six months prior to hospitalization. His parents reported that Steve had intermittently refused to go to school over the past two years due to somatic complaints, generalized panic, and strong fears of death. He was using drugs four to five times a week for the past one and one-half years. During this time, he spoke of homicidal and suicidal thoughts.

Until Steve was a fifth grader, he was described as a shy, but bright, sensitive, and adaptable child. Toward the end of the 5th grade, Steve was described as more hostile and insensitive to other children and was intermittently suspended from class.

Steve's father is a recovering alcoholic; he stopped drinking two years prior to Steve's hospitalization. Steve's role while his father was drinking was described as the mediator who offered support to both of his parents. His parents style of parenting was described as permissive and laissez faire, leaving Steve with a great deal of responsibility and autonomy at an early age.

Parent-Adolescent Group

During their first group, Steve and his parents had difficulty having a conversation or participating in any joint activity. Steve was sarcastic and negative toward any attempt that his parents made toward him. They gave up quickly and sat tensely and silently. Steve exhibited no interest in choosing an activity and seemed content to sit the group out. A leader structured the family into playing a game; the mood among them lightened somewhat, but little enjoyment of one another was observed.

The leaders' first goal was to first break the cycle of negative interaction by having Steve make an activity decision before his parents arrived. As Steve desired to return home and to live with his parents, he acknowledged that while in the hospital, he would participate in parent-adolescent group. He worked on a list of activities that were feasible and appropriate to engage in with his parents.

In the parents' pre-group, Steve's parents asked for ideas about possible ways to manage Steve when he became negative and withdrew from them. The leaders and other parents worked with them to analyze the pattern of interaction that occurred between them and Steve. Steve's parents then considered strategies for approaching Steve in activity and in conversation. In the parent adolescent group, the leaders modeled strategies when Steve and his parents became frustrated with one another.

Once engaged in the activity, both Steve and his parents continued to lighten and conversed around the activity. Some projects brought laughter and others an opportunity to compliment Steve or to express pride in their own contributions. Other projects presented challenges to individual family members' skills. With the help of the leaders, Steve and his parents managed the difficulties by problem solving out loud with each other. Over the course of a few weeks, Steve began to make plans for the next week's activities with his parents at the end of a group. As Steve's parents became more comfortable within the group and with interacting with Steve in activity, they began to use the group time to also discuss how they would spend time as a family when Steve went home on passes. The immediate pressure of needing to fill silence in their time together with conversation was diminished as the activity provided a focus and immediacy. Steve and his parents first talked about the activity at hand and over the course of the activity broached other topics as well.

Over the course of two months, both parents became more active in sharing their own interests with Steve and seeking out what interested him. Mrs. M. bought a model airplane for the family to work on in parent-adolescent group because she remembered Steve once liking to put together models. Mr. M. brought a backgammon set to share his love of the game with Steve. Steve rejected some of the ideas and activities that his parents suggested, but his parents' attempts opened a dialogue and a process of negotiation for joint family activity.

As Steve and his parents engaged in activity, the leaders engaged Steve and his family in discussing Steve's dreams and goals for his future. Like many adolescents, Steve had difficulty verbalizing what he wanted to do in the future. Through the discussion, his parents communicated that he was not alone and that he had their support.

Jill: Building a Relationship

Jill, a 17-year-old girl was admitted to an adolescent inpatient unit because she violated a PINS petition (Person In Need of Supervison) that her mother had filed. She was drinking to intoxication, smoked pot at least four days per week and was also cutting school. When she argued with her mother about these behaviors, she smashed her hands against the wall and struck her mother.

Jill was described as a shy and fearful child who dramatically changed when her parents divorced when she was 15. She changed peer groups to one that was involved in drug and alcohol abuse. She began staying out all night and missed so many classes that she failed the tenth grade.

During her first month of hospitalization, Jill's mother, Mrs. T., reported that she wanted to talk with Jill about her divorce and about the issues that she and Jill had as mother and daughter. Jill avoided talking with her mother and manipulated her mother into allowing her to go out with her boyfriend and friends instead of spending her pass time from the hospital with her family. Mrs. T expressed dissatisfaction with the quantity and quality of time that she spent with her daughter. She felt that they did not have a relationship beyond her providing Jill food and shelter. Mrs. T and Jill were referred to parent-adolescent group.

At their first group session, Jill was physically clingy toward her mother. She giggled and hung on her mother in a very childlike way. When a discussion was facilitated between them about possibilities for mutual activity, mother and daughter quickly became tense. They were not attuned to each other. Mrs. T. wanted to knit and crochet; Jill's facial expression and words made it clear that she would not participate in those activities. Jill voiced a desire to tie-dye; Mrs. T. stated that she couldn't imagine doing that activity. Jill's face tightened and she stood silently facing her mother. When a leader suggested that there might be other activities that Jill and her mother might enjoy together, Jill suggested making cookies to her mother; her mother acquiesced. Over the course of two months, Jill and her mother baked, worked with clay, made candy houses, and then tie-dyed.

In the pre-group, Mrs. T. spoke as a parent who wanted to reach out to her daughter as a parent, but in the parent-adolescent group, Mrs. T. was very dependent on her daughter for instruction and assistance. She also sought to have her ideas within projects take precedence over Jill's ideas. When Jill and Mrs. T made a candy house, Mrs. T. alternately criticized some of Jill's plans and offered up her ideas as stronger ones while depending on Jill to figure out how to implement her own ideas. In conversation, Mrs. T. autocratically told Jill what Jill would do differently post hospitalization. Jill openly responded with anger as she said that she was now being infantilized at 17. It was suggested that these issues about the rules with which Jill would need to abide be brought to family therapy meetings. Within parent-adolescent group, Jill and Mrs. T. were asked to explore a different part of their relationship through joint occupation and related conversation. In this way, they might forge a new relationship and better understand one another at their present stages of development.

After a few weeks of participating in more familiar cooking activities with Jill, Mrs. T agreed to tie-dye with Jill as Jill suggested in their first group. After completing one tie-dyed shirt with Jill, Mrs. T became visibly more engaged and enthusiastic about the activity. She insisted that they do the activity again so that she could make a shirt for herself. Jill was clear that she was not interested and was ready to do something different. Within the supportive environment of the group, Jill was successful in setting limits with her mother, but it was evident that it was difficult for Mrs. T. to stay attuned to her daughter's interests and to support her attempts at autonomous thinking.

In order to assist Mrs. T in working towards exhibiting more openness and interest in Jill's ideas, the leaders guided Mrs. T. in first meeting her own needs through independent activities. The leaders helped her to work parallel to Jill and to converse with Jill about their independent activities which included simple jewelry making and pottery. With facilitation from the leaders, Mrs. T. began to talk with Jill about making plans for Jill's future post high school. Jill seemed surprised by her mother's interest in her thoughts and discussed her desire to get into a program to become a hair stylist when she finished high school. Mrs. T. and Jill were able to have relaxed conversations in which Mrs. T. could offer support and encouragement to her daughter. Though they continued to have disagreements about household rules, they began to use leisure activity as a positive means to maintain communication and interaction.

William: Developing Independence

William, a 16-year-old boy diagnosed with Aspergers Syndrome, was admitted for severe behavior problems at home and in school. He made suicidal threats at home, and physically fought with peers in school.

In addition to his two parents, William's family included two brothers who attended college out of state. His parents, Mr. and Mrs. Peters, reported that William achieved developmental milestones as expected and developed typically until he was hospitalized for pneumonia at 15 months. Upon his return home, he developed head banging and an intolerance for being alone. In the second grade, he was reported to have severe difficulties with attention span and impulse control. At 11, he was hospitalized for depression. At 13, he developed severe obsessive-compulsive symptoms.

William was a shy, timid, and overly sensitive child who remained on the outskirts of his peer group. He expressed deep hurt about not feeling accepted or included by his peers in school. He was a gifted piano player, but exhibited mild motor coordination deficits in self care, school, and leisure activities, as well as Dyspraxia.

Initially, William was very dependent in parent-adolescent group. When he was challenged in an activity, William immediately demanded that his parents take over the task. He made no attempt to problem solve independently or attempt to work with his parents in solving a problem. Mrs. Peters automatically took over activities when she saw William exhibit even mild frustration. Each time, William whined that a task was too difficult, Mr. Peters physically tensed, told William to stop whining and to try to do the activity himself. Invariably, Mr. Peters quickly acquiesced and did whatever William demanded when William ignored his father's reprimand. This occurred frequently in the first four groups that the Peters attended. In what appeared to be a way to limit his interactions with William, Mr. Peters took out a newspaper out of his bag to read or excused himself and left the room for periods of time.

Though the Peters' own goal was to help William develop greater independence from them so that he could go to college and prepare for a career in music, they demonstrated no strategies for fostering William doing even simple tasks independently. For example, when William complained that his glasses were dirty, his father immediately took them and cleaned them. When a leader suggested that maybe William could clean his glasses himself, William refused and loudly repeated his demand. Only with the leaders setting limits, were the Peters able to withstand William's escalating anger at his parents not completing tasks for him and begin to foster William figuring out how to manage tasks independently or with minimal assistance. Throughout group sessions, a leader needed to question both William's routine of avoiding task challenges as well as the Peter's automatic response to any of his demands.

The primary focus for the Peters family in parent-adolescent group was to adjust the balance of their participation in family activities. Activities that interested William served as a medium to foster William's experimenting with shifting his very dependent stance with his parents to using his parents for support and assistance as needed. Prior to group sessions, William chose projects that he agreed to participate in along with his parents. He chose projects that he had learned to do individually or in other groups. In this way, he had a sense of familiarity and comfort with the activity and was more amenable to approaching the activities with his parents on a more equal footing and was more open to working out challenges within the task with the guidance of his parents and a leader.

On some tasks, William worked on one part of the project while his mother worked on another part. Besides teaching William's parents to step back and allow William to face simple challenges that he had the capacity to handle, the leaders taught Mr. and Mrs. Peters cognitive strategies for supporting William in solving problems as opposed to taking over projects for William. Over the course of a few months, William developed plans with his parents and the leaders for future family projects within the group. For example, as he discussed his favorite music and his goal of being a professional musician, he decided that he wanted to be a rock star for Halloween. He was invested in this idea and then took the lead role in brainstorming what he would need and what he would need to make in order to have a good costume.

As the Peters family worked on projects, the leaders facilitated conversation among them about William's leisure activities with other adolescents on the inpatient unit. William's ideas and interests were gently sought and he was helped to fully articulate his thoughts and ideas. From these discussions, Mr. and Mrs. Peters had an opportunity to hear about William's successful independent participation in activities with his peers and gained awareness that William had the potential for greater independence from them.

CONCLUSION

A parent-adolescent activity group was developed through adapting a group approach applied to younger children and their parents. The literature about the central factors that promote adolescent development within their families was applied to working with psychiatrically hospitalized adolescents and their families. The group used activity to promote parents' demonstration of support toward their adolescent offspring and to promote positive communication between parent and adolescent.

Using a parent-adolescent activity group intervention to assist families that include an adolescent with mental illness is not common occupational therapy practice. There is much potential for fostering stronger parent-child relationships in the interest of adolescents' occupational development toward adulthood. Further study is needed to analyze assessment and intervention methods for such a group.

REFERENCES

Allen, J. P. & Land, D. (1999). Attachment in adolescence. In J. Cassidy & P. R. Shaver (Eds.), *Handbook of Attachment: Theory, Research and Clinical Applications* (pp. 319-335). NY: Guilford Press.

Allen, J. P., McEthaney, K. B., Land, D. J., Kuperminc, G. P., Moore, C. W., O'Beirne-Kelly, H., & Kilmer, S. L. (2003). A secure base in adolescence: Markers of attachment security in the mother-adolescent relationship. *Child Development,* 74, 292-307.

Cafferty, H. & Leichtman, M. (2001). Facilitating the transition from residential treatment into the community: II Changing social work roles. *Residential Treatment for Children & Youth,* 19(2), 13-25.

Carson, J.L. & Parke, R. D. (1996) Reciprocal negative affect in parent-child interactions and children's peer competency. *Child Development,* 67, 2217-2226.

Grotevant, H. & Cooper, C. (1985). Patterns of interaction in family relationships and the development of identity exploration in adolescence, *Child Development,* 56, 415-428.

Gullotta, T. P., Adams, G. R., & Markstrom, C. A. (1999). *The Adolescent Experience.* 4th Ed. San Diego, CA: Academic Press.

Hauser, S., Vieyra, M. et al. (1985) Vulnerability and resilience in adolescence: Views from the family. *Journal of Early Adolescence,* 5, 81-100.

Leichtman, M. & Leichtman, M.L. (2001). Facilitating the transition from residential treatment into the community: I The Problem. *Residential Treatment for Children & Youth,* 19(1), 21-27.

McKeown, R.E., Garrison, C.Z., Jackson, K. L., Cuffe, S.P., Addy, C. L. & Waller, J. L. (1997). Family structure and cohesion and depressive symptoms in adolescents. *Journal of Research on Adolescence,* 7(3), 267-281.

Montemayor, R. (1983). Parents and adolescents in conflict: All families some of the time and some families most of the time. *Journal of Early Adolescence,* 3, 83-103.

Montemayor, R. (1986). Family variation in parent-adolescent storm and stress. *Journal of Adolescent Research,* 1, 15-31.

Pettit, G. S., Bates, J. E. & Dodge, K. A. (1997). Supportive parenting, ecological context, and children's adjustment: A seven-year longitudinal study. *Child Development,* 68, 908-923.

Shulman, S., Elicker, J., & Sroufe, L. A. (1994). Stages of friendship growth in preadolescence as related to attachment history. *Journal of Social and Personal Relationships,* 11, 341-361.

Slavson, S. R. & Schiffer, M. (1975). *Group Psychotherapies for Children: A Textbook.* NY: International Universities Press.

Steinberg, L. (1990). Autonomy, conflict, and harmony in the family relationship. In S. S. Felman & G. R. Elliott (Eds.), *At the threshold* (pp. 255-276). Cambridge, MA: Harvard University Press.

Teti, D. M. & Ablard, K. E. (1989). Security of attachment and infant-sibling relationships: A laboratory study. *Child Development,* 60, 1519-1528.

Zabriskie, R. B. & McCormick, B. P. (2003). Parent and child perspectives of family leisure involvement and satisfaction with family life. *Journal of Leisure Research,* 32(2), 163-189.

doi:10.1300/J004v22n03_08

Chapter 9

When a Mother Is Depressed:
Supporting Her Capacity to Participate
in Co-Occupation with Her Baby–
A Case Study

SUMMARY. The literature related to mother-child interaction when a mother is depressed and a framework for addressing mother-child co-occupations for mothers with depression and their young children is provided. An in-depth case example that spans mother-infant occupation- based intervention during a short-term psychiatric hospitalization through home-based occupation-based intervention is provided. doi:10.1300/J004v22n03_09 *[Article copies available for a fee from The Haworth Document Delivery Service: 1-800-HAWORTH. E-mail address: <docdelivery@ haworthpress.com> Website: <http://www.HaworthPress.com> © 2006 by The Haworth Press, Inc. All rights reserved.]*

KEYWORDS. Parental depression, mother-child intervention, occupational therapy

In this chapter, I will describe what I did as an occupational therapist working at a large private psychiatric teaching hospital to address the

---

[Haworth co-indexing entry note]: "When a Mother Is Depressed: Supporting Her Capacity to Participate in Co-Occupation with Her Baby–A Case Study." Olson, Laurette. Co-published simultaneously in *Occupational Therapy in Mental Health* (The Haworth Press, Inc.) Vol. 22, No. 3/4, 2006, pp. 135-152; and: *Activity Groups in Family-Centered Treatment: Psychiatric Occupational Therapy Approaches for Parents and Children* (Laurette Olson) The Haworth Press, Inc., 2006, pp. 135-152. Single or multiple copies of this article are available for a fee from The Haworth Document Delivery Service [1-800- HAWORTH, 9:00 a.m. - 5:00 p.m. (EST). E-mail address: docdelivery@haworthpress.com].

needs of one mother with mental illness and her baby. My goal is to provide an example of one way that occupational therapists may use their skills beyond their traditional roles on inpatient psychiatric units and as home-based service providers to assist parents with mental illness more successfully parent.

Eileen was a young woman diagnosed with depression who identified working on parenting her nine-month-old baby boy, Michael, as her key rehabilitation goal. My assessment and intervention methods were based upon psychiatric rehabilitation, cognitive-behavioral therapy and a parent-child activity therapy approach that I had previously developed. I will first share literature about parental depression and its impact on parent-child relationships and will then describe my framework for providing occupational therapy for depressed parents and their children.

I began my work with Eileen at the end of her first week of a one month psychiatric hospitalization. Eileen and I had six sessions with her baby over the course of the remaining three weeks of her hospitalization. Upon the psychiatric team's recommendation and Eileen's request for continued parent-child occupation based intervention, I continued my work with her with her in home for two more years. Eileen's husband and her parents intermittently participated in our work as they were also Michael's caregivers and supported Eileen as she worked to participate as fully as possible in parenting Michael.

LITERATURE RELATED TO MATERNAL DEPRESSION

Downey and Coyne (1990) analyzed research that suggests that depressed parents' interactions with their children resemble their behaviors with adults. Depressed parents speak less often and with less intensity, gaze less frequently at their children, respond less positively, less frequently and more slowly to their children's attempts to engage them. Hops et al. (1987) studied depressed and non-depressed mothers and their families in their homes and found that depressed mothers behave in ways that are more aversive to children than typical mothers do, in addition to not providing positive reinforcement for their children which may be aversive in itself. Radke-Yarrow, Nottelman, Belmont, and Welsh (1993) also found that depressed mothers expressed significantly more negative affect than did mothers who were not diagnosed as depressed. Bandura et al. (2003) reported that affect can have a generalized impact on a person's sense of self efficacy. An intense negative affect can reduce one's sense of self efficacy and engagement in tasks. One might expect that a mother with depression might therefore be likely to perceive herself negatively as a mother and engage less frequently in parenting tasks than other mothers might.

Downey and Coyne (1990) reported that as early as three months, infants of depressed mothers reciprocate their mother's negative and less effortful interactive behavior. Downey and Coyne (1990) also reported that available evidence suggests that the adjustment of children does not improve as a mother's depression lessens. They suggested that there is likely chronic impairment and family stress that occur with parental depression.

Parents and children may have developed negative beliefs and expectations about each other over the course of parents' depression and may continue to enter new parent-child interactions with the expectation of a negative or unhelpful response. Because expectations influence behavior, it is likely that parents and children may avoid one another or respond to each other in a manner consistent with their expectations. Over time, a negative interaction cycle may become habitual. During a parent's depression, children may avoid their parents and come to expect that their parent would be easily upset or irritated by their requests or behavior. They may expect that their parent will not be able to help them with homework or everyday problems. Parents with depression may find themselves emotionally removed from family activity and be uninvolved in their children's everyday life. Even after they receive medical treatment for their depression, they may find it difficult and overwhelming to re-enter activities with their children.

To develop more positive and productive interaction patterns, parents and children may need to have different experiences with each other and be guided in altering the habitual patterns of interacting that developed during a parent's depression. Though repairing relationships with their children who may have experienced neglect or rejection during their depression may be very challenging for a parent, it is critical for the emotional development and well-being of their children, as well as for their own self efficacy in their life role as a parent.

Studies of typical families have consistently correlated positive parent-child relationships with children's competence in others areas of functioning, such as resourcefulness (Arend, Gove, & Sroufe, 1979), problem solving skills (Matas, Arend, & Sroufe, 1978), coping skills (Murphy, 1967), and good peer relationships (Lieberman, 1977; Waters, Wippman, & Sroufe, 1979). Murphy (1967) examined characteristics of the mother-child relationship that appear to help or hinder a child's development of coping skills. Murphy found that the most important variables are the quality of a mother's enjoyment, active support, and encouragement of her child. The research of Eisenberg et al. (2003) suggests that maternal expression of positive emotion is related to children's social competence and adjustment. Pettit, Bates, and Dodge (1997) found that supportive parenting (mother to child warmth, proactive teaching, inductive discipline and positive involvement) is positively linked with children's adjustment including social skills, academic performance and behavior even in the face of family adversity. Depressed mothers are likely to have difficulty offering sufficient and consistent support, instrumental assistance and expression of positive emotion to their offspring and more likely to express negative emotion. Toddlers who experienced high levels of maternal negativity were found to be more likely to exhibit behavior problems two years later (Rubin, Burgess, Dwyer, & Hastings, 2003).

There are some studies examining ways of increasing the ability of depressed women to have more positive parent-child relationships with their children. Stott et al. (1984) suggested that parents who experienced direct intervention that also included their children might be more in tune with their children than parents who only receive counseling.

The results of the 1989 study by Jouriles, Murphy, and O'Leary suggest that maternal mood influences maternal interactions with preschool age children. During a negative mood condition, mothers issued fewer positive statements toward their children and engaged in less verbal interaction; reciprocally children were less compliant with their mothers than they were during a positive mood condition. A 1989 study by Lay, Waters, and Park suggests that responsive play increases positive mood, and that children who were induced into positive moods were more compliant and complied in shorter periods of time than children induced into negative moods. These findings are consistent with the work of Bandura et al. (2003) who suggest that positive affect supports activity engagement.

Though there are not any published studies by occupational therapists related to examining how to support the optimal functioning of depressed mothers and their children, it is a critical topic that should be addressed. Occupational therapists work with children and adults and their families in medical, rehabilitative, educational, community, and private practice settings. The mandate for occupational therapists is to improve the everyday functioning of their clients in their daily life roles. Parental depression is not unusual in any practice setting, but it is rarely addressed directly by occupational therapists. It is important that occupational therapists work with interdisciplinary teams to assess the ability of depressed parents and their children to positively interact with each other in everyday parent-child activities that support children's development and participation in their daily occupations, as well as support parents' sense of personal self efficacy as caregivers. Occupational therapists can create a therapeutic environment that helps parents and children to experience one another positively and supports their development of skills necessary to successfully participate in their joint family occupations.

To help depressed parents develop the skills to positively engage their children in everyday activities, I developed guidelines for parent-child activity intervention to address the particular issues that these parents may exhibit which limit their success in developing a positive parent-child relationship. My guidelines are based upon my understanding of the literature related to mothers with depression, behavioral, and cognitive behavior therapy, as well as on my previous work providing parent-child activity intervention for families that included children with mental illness.

APPLYING CONCEPTS
OF COGNITIVE BEHAVIORAL THERAPY

When a mother competently participates in a mutually enjoyable activity with her child, she is positively reinforced by the smiles of her child, the affection engendered between them and the concrete results of the task. Consequently this increases the likelihood that she will actively participate in similar mother-child activities in the future.

In mother-child interactions, depressed mothers have been found to have difficulty sustaining task focus, to be more self-focused, less active, expect and express less pleasure, respond more negatively, less frequently and more slowly to their children's attempts to engage them (Gotlib & Hammen, 1992; Downey & Coyne, 1990). These changes in cognition and behaviors noted in mothers with depression interfere with their ability to act in ways that will be positively reinforcing to their children or that they will be reinforced by positive behavior displayed by their children. Decreased positive reinforcement further increases self-focused attention (Lewinshohn, Hoberman, Teri, & Hautzinger, 1985).

Self-focused attention is a cognitive state in which one selectively attends to information that originates from within and concerns the self (Carver & Scheier, 1981). In this state, a person is more aware of discrepancies between the behavior of the ideal self and one's actual behavior and is therefore, more self critical. Affective reactions are intensified, awareness of anxiety increases and frustration with tasks results in an increased likelihood to withdraw from challenges (Lewinsohn et al., 1985). When self-focused attention is coupled with negative expectations as is typical in persons with depression, effort and persistence significantly decrease (Carver & Scheier, 1981).

A person is likely to rapidly attend to and participate in an activity that is positively reinforcing. If experiences of pleasure in mother-child activity increase, it is most likely that a depressed mother will open to participating in similar activities with her children. This outward focus will lessen the amount of self focus. With multiple experiences of pleasure in activity, she will likely begin to expect pleasure in similar circumstances in the future. Positive expectations will make it more likely that she will attend and exhibit effort in these mother-child activities.

The challenge for the therapist is to create an occupational environment and to choose activities that will initially engage a mother who may have difficulty sustaining task focus, be inwardly focused, have negative expectations, be passive and slow to respond with her child in a joint activity. The therapist initially takes responsibility for the setting up of the environment and activity and for facilitating positive parent-child activity interaction. The therapist then arranges additional similar opportunities for positive interaction so that parent and child expect certain joint activities to be pleasurable.

Once a mother expects that some interactions can be manageable and positive, the therapist engages her in setting up the environment or choosing activities for mother-child sessions so that she becomes aware that she can exhibit a degree of self control over environmental conditions. She can change part of the environment that feels uncomfortable or negative to her. She can also positively affect her mood by adding elements to the environment that feel relaxing, organizing, or energizing to her and her child. This may include limiting extraneous noise, playing background music, clearing the room of distractions, or asking her spouse to be present. The therapist then addresses managing challenges and conflicts within the activity process between parent and child.

Specific guidelines for supporting a depressed mother to engage with her child are:

1. If the therapist sets up an activity so that a mother and child have the cognitive and motor capacity to successfully participate and

that both find pleasurable and then facilitates the activity process, the mother will likely exhibit behaviors suggesting reduced self-focused attention.

2. If a mother has multiple experiences of pleasurable and successful activity interactions with her child in a supportive environment, she will begin to expect success with similar activities in that environment.

3. If a mother has multiple experiences of successfully managing disruptions or challenges in the activity process with her child in a supportive environment, she will begin to expect that disruptions and challenges are manageable in that environment.

4. When a mother experiences consistent success and pleasure in activities with her child in a supportive environment, she will likely be open to planning independent parent-child activities that she and her child will do in her home or community environment.

5. If a mother is assisted in applying/adapting techniques used in therapy sessions to manage challenges and disruptions in activity interactions at home, she will likely expect success in using these techniques in activity with her child.

6. If a mother can identify how environment or environmental conditions affect her mood state and how this affects her mother-child interaction, she will likely be open to manipulating the environment or environmental conditions to support positive parent-child activity interaction.

CASE DESCRIPTION

The setting where I worked with Eileen and her baby during her short term psychiatric hospitalization was a large private psychiatric teaching hospital where the rehabilitation department (including occupational therapists, rehabilitation counselors, recreational and creative arts therapists) adopted the psychiatric rehabilitation philosophy and practice guidelines for its work with all patients. According to the psychiatric rehabilitation framework (Anthony, Cohen, Farkas, & Gayne, 2002), persons with mental illness need to be equal partners with therapists in their own rehabilitation including identifying what their rehabilitation needs and goals are. Clients identify where they would like to live and what they would like to be doing within a few months. Therapists then work with clients to articulate the critical skills needed to achieve the clients' goals for living and working within their desired environments. The psychiatric rehabilitation philosophy is consistent with best practice in occupational therapy. Occupational therapists strive to help their clients optimally participate in their present occupations and develop the skills and adapt or alter the tasks or environments to support clients' participation in their desired occupations and related tasks.

During initial interviews, therapists sought to learn what patients wanted to do and where they wanted to live post hospitalization. A cluster of patients identified wanting to go home to parent their children. They identified improving their parenting skills and developing a strong positive relationship with their children as critical skills that they needed to address during their hospitalization. Eileen, a young mother of a nine-month-old baby, was one of these patients.

Eileen, a young woman in her early thirties, had been happily married and had a successful career in a major corporation in a major metropolitan area. She and her husband, Mike, owned a home in a suburb and enjoyed decorating and maintaining the home, as well as entertaining their extended families and friends.

When Eileen became pregnant, memories of being sexually abused as a young adolescent flooded her mind. Despite having a supportive husband, family and friends who rejoiced in her pregnancy, Eileen wanted to terminate her pregnancy. Eileen reported that prior to her pregnancy, she always enjoyed children and was considered an excellent caregiver to her nieces and nephews. Eileen acquiesced to the pressure of her husband, family and friends and carried her baby to full term.

Throughout her pregnancy, Eileen saw her psychotherapist weekly to help her manage her feelings and emotions about her past sexual abuse and about becoming a mother. Her distress further increased when she discovered that she would be the mother of a boy. Eileen informed her psychiatrist and family that she thought it was best to give up her son for adoption immediately after his birth. Her husband and family vehemently opposed this. Eileen gave birth to a healthy infant and went home with her infant son, Michael, a few days after his birth. She expressed little interest in seeing or caring for him in the hospital, but her husband and family assumed that she would adjust to motherhood once she was at home. At home, Eileen became more distraught as she was left alone with her infant. Eileen's parents quickly rearranged their daily schedule to visit Eileen to assist her in caring for their grandson. Eileen remained emotionally and physically removed from her son. She did not participate in any care-giving tasks when other caregivers were present.

Within a few months, Eileen tried to kill herself and was hospitalized on an acute psychiatric unit. She participated in individual and group therapy, received medication and her impulses to kill herself subsided. She was discharged after a month, but was re-hospitalized a few months later due to a second suicide attempt.

I met Eileen one week after her second psychiatric admission. Eileen reported that she felt that her treatment during her first psychiatric hospitalization was ineffective because her baby was not part of her treatment. Eileen identified that her primary goal for this hospitalization was to learn to mother her baby. She stated that not being able to mother Michael was the reason that she attempted suicide and could not participate in any other life occupations. She stated that she would likely feel suicidal again unless she was able to mother her child.

Eileen reported that not being able to hold her baby or care for him in any way was causing her a great deal of pain, in addition to being very upsetting to her husband and family. She also stated that she knew that her inability to nurture her baby was harmful to him physically and psychologically. After Eileen and I met and developed a plan for occupational therapy sessions that included her baby, Eileen elicited the assistance of her parents and husband to get her nine-month-old son, Michael, to the hospital for parent-child occupational therapy sessions two times per week.

While Eileen was very focused on increasing her comfort with holding and caring for her infant son, she also held strong beliefs that her baby would be controlling of her through his demands for attention. Her expectations colored all of her interactions with Michael. Changing her beliefs about Michael was equally as important as creating an environment where Eileen could experience her interactions with Michael as engaging and manageable.

Parent-Child Occupational Based Treatment as Part of a Short-Term Hospitalization

Eileen was inwardly focused, very anxious about interacting with her baby, avoided eye contact with him and preferred to watch others hold and care for him. She had very low expectations that she would be able to successfully or pleasurably engage her baby. In the presence of her baby, she could remain focused on him only briefly before stating that she felt overwhelmed and anxious. When Eileen handled her son, she made no eye contact and exhibited a bland affect. Michael did not spontaneously seek her when she entered the room; he was content with his grandparents and sought them out for play and interaction.

Eileen's six occupational therapy sessions during her three week hospitalization focused on facilitating Eileen's engagement in a few central tasks important for developing a mother-child relationship with her nine-month-old baby. Before her first two sessions, an environment for play and interaction was set up prior to the arrival of Eileen and her baby. In spite of her stated desire to learn to parent Michael, Eileen's expectation of being overwhelmed by her child was so great that she needed gentle coaching and support to approach and touch Michael.

In our first session, Eileen hesitantly sat next to her mother, looked and gently touched her baby. I first engaged Michael by smiling and making faces at him; he smiled and laughed. I gently asked Eileen to try as well. She then tentatively moved her face closer to him and gently smiled at him. When he returned her smile and she continued to playfully gaze at him. We moved him to the floor so that Michael could freely play with his toys as well as be able to interact with his mother. Eileen tentatively picked him up and put him on a blanket that she and I had set up with two toys on it. I initiated play with Michael and then engaged Eileen in the play with Michael and me. Eileen pulled back after brief interchanges with Michael. With support, she attracted Michael to play with her by engaging with one of his toys along with him. She expressed enjoying her brief interchanges with Michael, but described feeling very stressed by it as well. She stated that she was afraid that if she played with her son, he would make increasing demands of her.

In each session, I engaged Eileen and Michael with each other in play activities that interested Michael and were comfortable for Eileen. After our second session, Eileen helped to set up the space for parent-child sessions and discussed with me how we would use our hour long session. Before each session, Eileen also talked with her parents about toys that they might bring that she might use to engage Michael with her. In each session, play was used to engage Eileen with her son, alter her mood and increase her outward focus as well as increase her son's attention and comfort with her. Following play, care-giving activities that were important to Michael's basic care were carried out. Eileen changed his clothing and diaper, prepared a bottle and snack for her son. Eileen had the underlying cognitive and task skills to perform these tasks. She lacked the initiative to carry out these routine care-giving activities. Each session concluded with a discussion of Eileen's subjective experience of her interactions with her son within the session.

During her hospitalization, Eileen began to hold, feed and play with Michael for up to 45 minutes per session. She also became increasingly aware of how her fears of her son limited her ability to relax and fully enjoy him. She also became conscious of how she used other activities as excuses to limit interaction with him.

At discharge, Eileen stated that she was feeling better because she was now able to positively interact with her baby within her parent-child therapy sessions, but was concerned about how she would manage at home. Though Eileen's parents agreed to care for their grandson during the week until Eileen and her husband, Jason, were ready to be full time parents, Eileen was fearful that she would not be able to mother her son each weekend.

To support Eileen's continued recovery post hospitalization and to reduce the likelihood of re-hospitalization, it was recommended that Eileen continue to receive parent-child occupation based services as an outpatient. I recommended that these services be home-based so that I could observe how she participated in activities with her child in her home. In this way, we could identify the central skills that she needed to develop and adapt tasks and her home environment to support her ability to co-parent her child with her husband.

Home-Based Parent Child Occupational Therapy Sessions

Eileen received home-based parent-child occupational therapy services one time per week in addition to outpatient psychotherapy for two years. Occupational therapy sessions occurred weekly on Sunday mornings, the second day that Eileen and Jason had their son at home with them. In this way, in addition to promoting positive occupational engagement within Eileen's home environment, events of the previous day could be discussed and plans for second day could made in light of what had previously occurred. There were also opportunities to analyze the set up of the home and daily routines for safe and productive daily living for parents and child.

During weekends, Jason was the primary caregiver. Eileen gradually took responsibility for the care of Michael for increasing lengths of time. During agreed upon periods of time, Jason worked in another part of the house while Eileen took charge of Michael. He was close enough so that Eileen could call him if she felt that she needed help with Michael. Jason could also monitor Eileen and Michael's interaction from a distance and step in if necessary.

Both Eileen's parents and Jason were intermittently engaged in Eileen's home based parent child sessions so that they would better understand the nature of the parent-child intervention and be supportive of Eileen as she applied what she worked on in sessions. They also provided Eileen feedback on their perceptions of Michael's behavior and Eileen's interaction with Michael so that Eileen and I could compare with her own perceptions. Throughout Eileen's parent-child occupational therapy intervention, I had regular phone contact with Eileen's psychiatrist so that my work complemented and supported Eileen's overall psychiatric outpatient treatment.

Though Eileen made excellent gains in playing and caring for her child within occupational therapy sessions within an inpatient psychiatric environment, her home was a more challenging context and the progress that she made was very fragile. Within her home, she was distracted by other tasks that interested her more and helped her avoid her baby. She also described how easy it would be to fall back into her routine prior to her hospitalization. A new routine for living with her husband and baby needed to be established.

Eileen's home was not arranged for a baby to play safely and there were many items that were important to Eileen that were in easy reach for a growing child. Eileen initially resisted any recommendations to alter her home environment as she associated this with more demands that interfered with her own wishes and controlled her. Her views were challenged as she and I observed and played with her child in her home. A cognitive approach was used to analyze how she wanted her baby to behave and what she valued as a mother compared to what actually was occurring.

Providing services within Eileen's home environment offered Eileen opportunities to transfer learning from the hospital environment to her everyday interactions with Michael at home. In our first sessions, Eileen reported that Michael was a poor eater in her home, in spite of being a very good eater at her mother's home. I observed Eileen set up her kitchen to feed Michael and analyzed what interfered with Michael attending to her and the task of eating. What I observed was that it was difficult for her to remain focused on her child as she fed him. She was preoccupied with other tasks that she wanted to do within her home and was easily distracted. Eileen didn't keep Michael engaged in the co-occupation of feeding, missed his cues and therefore wasn't aware of the possibility to adjust her style or speed of feeding to better engage her son. Michael was also easily distracted and rapidly became fussy while Eileen quickly became frustrated.

Eileen and I set up the corner of her kitchen where she sat Michael for meals so that she and Michael would be less visually distracted, more relaxed and be more likely to focus on one another. One of our first goals was to increase Eileen's awareness of Michael's behavioral cues as she fed him so that she had the opportunity to respond effectively and remain in control of the activity.

Feeding and engaging Michael over breakfast became a key activity for our sessions over our two years of home-based occupational therapy sessions. Feeding issues changed as Michael grew. Tolerating less than perfect self-feeding was difficult for Eileen and we worked on fostering Michael's independence in feeding himself by exploring the types of food that were healthy, he enjoyed and she could tolerate Michael feeding himself.

As a preschooler, Michael was at times resistive in coming to the table because he didn't want to leave a play activity. Eileen's communication to Michael prior to breakfast was often confusing. For example, one morning as she was almost finished fixing breakfast, Eileen said, "Michael, do you want to go downstairs to play?" Michael happily complied and within five minutes, Eileen requested that he come up for breakfast. Michael had a temper tantrum as he had just become involved in play. Sessions focused on setting up a routine so that Michael could anticipate what would occur next as well as on ways to engage Michael to make transitions from play to meals. The routines that we set up for Michael were also supportive to Eileen's capacity to mother.

Promoting Parent-Child Play

A key vehicle to connect to one's children is parent-child play and leisure interaction. Through play, children relax and focus on their own terms and create a separate cognitive and emotional space from the space that they inhabit in the rest of their daily lives with adults. When parents have the capacity to play with their children, they are afforded the opportunity to relate to their children in a different way than they typically do in daily care-giving interactions. Within play, children express their thoughts, feeling and wishes about events in their lives and also work to understand and meet the challenges inherent in mastering objects and materials and activities of interest. Parents have the opportunity to gain insight into their children's ways of thinking about and interacting with objects and people.

In order to play with another, one must not only approach another in a relaxed and open manner, but also get "in step" with that person. A player observes and reads the nonverbal cues of a playmate and adapts personal play goals in consideration of the goals and approaches of the other. Two people meet on common ground in play.

When adults interact with children, they typically control the situation by providing structure, limits and guidance as necessary in the interest of insuring children's survival and growth. Children most often follow the rules and directions of adults to maintain strong relationships with their care providers. Adults' inherent power over children can impede children's ability to engage in play with adults unless adults work to enter children's play world and follow children's cues.

Eileen not only had difficulty engaging Michael in a relaxed and open manner, but she also tended to disrupt his play by introducing ideas for activity that were not in synchrony with his own play direction, distracted him from his play, or were beyond his developmental capacities. For example, as Eileen watched Michael attempt to make a moon out of Playdoh™, she attempted to draw Michael's attention by putting a piece of Playdoh™ on her nose. He did the same and soon had Playdoh™ in his mouth. During another session, she suggested that he mold the Playdoh™ to make a face like she was forming out of the clay. Her sculpture was detailed and far beyond what Michael was capable of producing. He quickly withdrew from the activity stating that it was too hard to make things.

Over a two year period, we worked on developing her capacity to engage in play with her son. Each week, we set up an environment for play including developmentally engaging toys and materials that were consonant with Michael's interests and skill levels. We examined the household areas where Michael played and figured out ways to set them up for Michael that were also acceptable to her. We observed Michael play, worked to read his cues and participated in his play.

Learning to tolerate Michael's expressions of frustration when a construction fell down or pieces of his train fell apart so that he would learn how to cope with simple challenges in play was difficult for Eileen. She identified with his frustration as well as was irritated by his whining; she had the impulse to quickly fix the situation or withdraw from the room. Eileen first reflected on her own identification and feelings about what she observed in her son. As she read about supporting children's coping skills and practiced offering quiet emotional support, practical assistance, or additional structure or limits to support her son's coping efforts, she also reflected upon her own coping skills as a mother.

At 2, Michael exhibited a special interest in music and in playing the family piano that mirrored his mother's love of music. Playing the piano was used as an activity through which Eileen could engage Michael in joint activity and an activity in which Michael would most likely prefer his mother's participation over other caregivers. Eileen was physically more relaxed and expressive at the piano than she was participating in other activities with her son. Reciprocally, Michael was focused and exhibited much pleasure in the activity and in his mother. Eileen enjoyed showing him simple sequences of musical sounds, Michael was attentive when she demonstrated and taught him how to play simple musical sequences. His behavior was as positively reinforcing to her, as her attention was to him.

Planning Daily Occupation-Based Activities

In addition to my concrete work helping Eileen engage in her daily occupations with Michael, we also worked on planning activities related to mother-child co-occupations that occurred at other times. We brainstormed activities that she might independently participate with her child outside of sessions and then narrowed down the list to those activities that she thought that she would likely succeed in engaging Michael. We then planned and carried out some of those activities in our sessions to explore how well Michael would receive them and to explore potential challenges that would be inherent in carrying out these and similar activities.

When Michael was three, Eileen wanted to decorate a Halloween pumpkin with Michael. Eileen originally decided that she wanted to cut out a pumpkin with Michael and then decorate it. Eileen bought a pumpkin and we tried cutting out a pumpkin and Eileen saw that cutting was well beyond the skill and interest of her son. We also had ripped paper, yarn and markers available and Eileen learned that Michael was very interested in decorating his pumpkin with these supplies.

An issue uncovered in our discussions during our home-based work was the difficulty taking Michael to family events. Other family members typically remembered items that were important for managing young children; they did not expect Eileen to remember. Eileen was aware that others were viewing her as incompetent and felt sorry for her as a mother who was recently psychiatrically hospitalized. Eileen wanted to be in charge of her child and be viewed as prepared and competent as other mothers. We made lists of what she would need to pack so that she would be able to appropriately care for and entertain Michael at family events. We worked on anticipating what taking her son to a christening would be like and what she would need to do to set up a positive structure for Michael. Eileen prepared a bag with a small snack and small toys to entertain her son in church as well as wipes and materials to wash him and change him. Her experience of self efficacy after having succeeded at the first family event opened the door to her wanting to plan and prepare for other events including planning local trips to the park and zoo.

Becoming Aware of the Impact of Depressive Symptoms on Everyday Parenting

The relationship of effectively managing the symptoms of her depression and her ability to carry out the central tasks of parenting became clear to Eileen in our discussions of her daily occupation of mothering Michael. In one session, Eileen said:

> I don't know. . . I sometimes think, oh, he's all right. . . so he's wet. . . If I change him, he'll just get wet again. . . He's all right playing on the stairs. If he falls, he'll learn not to do it again. . .

She became more aware and then concerned about her thoughts that minimized Michael's physical discomforts or potential dangers. As we compared her behavior at these times to her behavior at other times, she acknowledged changes in her routines that included irregularly taking her medication and having difficulty getting out of bed. With greater awareness about the impact of symptoms of depression on her capacity to mother, she called her psychiatrist to have her medication adjusted. In collaboration with her husband, she worked out a concrete plan to remember to take her medications.

Once Michael grew to be a toddler, like many toddlers, he explored all items within his reach. He accidentally broke household items such as a favorite dish and mug. One of Eileen's initial responses to Michael was, "You, stupid jerk. . . get out of here, I don't want anything to do with you!" She became so upset that she refused to have him in the same room. She stated that she wanted her child to feel pain and she withdrew to her bed. Within our sessions, Eileen confronted the mismatch between her overwhelming anger about the incidents and the actual facts of the incidents. We examined the physical environment and the players involved in each incident. In order to explore what happened, we set up the environment as it likely was, re-enacted the situation and then rearranged the environment to reduce Michael's opportunity to touch her personal things and then imagine a different outcome. We read and discussed books that explained and outlined how to apply cognitive strategies to everyday life such as *The Feeling Good Handbook* and *Learned Optimism*. We also read and practiced effective limit setting strategies for a child Michael's age.

CONCLUSION

In this chapter, I highlighted what occupational therapy added to the psychosocial intervention for a young mother with depression. Other professionals played central roles in her inpatient psychiatric treatment and outpatient therapy. I mentioned their work only briefly because the work of other mental health professionals is well documented. There is very sparse literature suggesting that occupational therapy can play a key role in mental health interventions with mothers who are depressed. It is important that ways in which occupational therapists have contributed to helping mothers with depression participate in their co-occupations with their children be documented and that potential fruitful approaches for this work be articulated. I hope that my description of my work with Eileen and her baby resonates with the experiences of other occupational therapists working with mothers diagnosed with depression and their babies and facilitates their thinking more deeply about optimal occupation-based mother-child interventions. Possibly, therapists who have not considered intervening in mother-child co-occupation with mothers exhibiting symptoms of depression and their babies might reflect on ways to support mothers like Eileen whom they might meet within their occupational therapy practice.

REFERENCES

Anthony, W.A., Cohen, M.R., Farkas, M.D., & Gagne, C. (2002). *Psychiatric Rehabilitation, 2nd edition*. Boston, MA: Boston University, Center for Psychiatric Rehabilitation.

Arend, R., Gove, F.L., & Sroufe, L. A. (1979). Continuity of individual adaptation from infancy to kindergarten: A predictive study of ego resilience and curiosity in preschoolers. *Child Development, 50*, 950-957.

Bandura, A., Caprara, G. V., Barbaranelli, C., Gerbino, M., & Pastorelli, C. (2003). Role of affective self-regulatory efficacy in diverse spheres of psychosocial functioning. *Child Development, 74* (3), 769-782.

Burns, D. D. (1990). *The Feeling Good Handbook*. NY: Penguin

Carver, C.S. & Scheier, M. F. (1981). *Attention and Self Regulation: A Control Theory Approach to Human Behavior.* New York: Springer-Verlag.

Dodge, K.A. (1990). Developmental psychopathology in children of depressed mothers. *Developmental Psychology,* 26, 3-6.

Downey, G. & Coyne, J. C. (1990). Children of depressed parents: An integrative review. *Psychological Bulletin,* 108, 50-76.

Eisenberg, N., Valiente, C., Morris, A.S., Fabes, R. A., Cumberland, A., & Reiser, M. et al. (2003) Longitudinal relations among parental emotional expressivity, children's regulations and quality of socioemotional functioning. *Developmental Psychology,* 39, 3-19.

Field, T. (1998). Emotional care of the at risk infant: Early interventions for infants of depressed mothers. *Pediatrics,* 102(5) Supplement, Nov. 1998 1305-1310.

Jouriles, E. N., Murphy, C. M., & O'Leary, K. D. (1989). Effects of maternal mood on mother-son interaction patterns. *Journal of Abnormal Child Psychology,* 17, 513-525.

Lay, K., Waters, E., & Park, K. (1989). Maternal responsiveness and child compliance: The role of mood as a mediator, *Child Development,* 60, 1405-1411.

Lewinshohn, P. M., Hoberman, H. M., Teri, L., & Hautzinger, M. (1985). An integrative theory of depression. In S. Reiss & R.R. Bootzin (Eds). *Theoretical Issues in Behavior Therapy.* London: Academic Press, Inc.

Lieberman, A. F. (1977). Preschoolers' competence with a peer: Influence of attachment and social experience. *Child Development,* 48, 1277-1287.

Matas, L., Arend, R., & Sroufe, L. A. (1978). Continuity of adaptation in the second year: The relationship of the quality of attachment and later competence. *Child Development,* 24, 65-81.

Nicholson, J. & Henry, A. D. (2003). Achieving the goal of evidence-based psychiatric rehabilitation practices for mothers with mental illnesses. *Psychiatric Rehabilitation Journal,* 27, 122-130.

Oyserman, D., Mawbray, C. T., Meares, P. A., & Firminger, K. B. (2000). Parenting among mothers with a serious mental illness. *American Journal of Orthopsychiatry,* 70(3), 296-315.

Pettit, G. S., Bates, J. E. & Dodge, K. A. (1997). Supportive parenting, ecological context, and children's adjustment: A seven-year longitudinal study. *Child Development,* 68, 908-923.

Rubin, K. H., Burgess, K. B., Dwyer, K. M., & Hastings, P. D. (2003). Predicting preschoolers' externalizing behaviors from toddler temperament, conflict, and maternal negativity. *Developmental Psychology,* 39, 164-176.

Seligman, M. E. P. (1991). *Learned Optimism.* NY: Knopf.

Teti, D. M. & Gelfand, D. M. (1991). Behavioral competence among mothers of infants in the first year: The mediational role of maternal self-efficacy. *Child Development,* 62, 918-929.

Waters, E., Wippman, J., & Sroufe, L. Q. (1979). Attachment, positive affect and competence in the peer group: Two studies in construct validation. *Child Development,* 50, 821-829.

Weinberg, M. K. & Tronick, E. Z. (1998). Emotional care of the at-risk infant: Emotional characteristics of infants associated with maternal depression and anxiety. *Pediatrics,* 102(2) Supplement, Nov. 1998, 1298-1304.

doi:10.1300/J004v22n03_09

Chapter 10

Closing Thoughts About Promoting Parent-Child Co-Occupation Through Parent-Child Activity Intervention

SUMMARY. Parent-child and parent-adolescent activity groups and parent-child occupation-based intervention meet different mental health needs and provide a different service than what is typically offered in a psychiatric setting. These interventions are designed to promote and/or develop positive interactions and engagement between parents and children in co-occupations. doi:10.1300/J004v22n03_10 *[Article copies available for a fee from The Haworth Document Delivery Service: 1-800-HAWORTH. E-mail address: <docdelivery@haworthpress.com> Website: <http://www.HaworthPress.com> © 2006 by The Haworth Press, Inc. All rights reserved.]*

KEYWORDS. Occupational therapy, families, mental illness

My qualitative research expands the therapeutic approach to assisting parents and their psychiatrically hospitalized children in establish-

[Haworth co-indexing entry note]: "Closing Thoughts About Promoting Parent-Child Co-Occupation Through Parent-Child Activity Intervention." Olson, Laurette. Co-published simultaneously in *Occupational Therapy in Mental Health* (The Haworth Press, Inc.) Vol. 22, No. 3/4, 2006, pp. 153-156; and: *Activity Groups in Family-Centered Treatment: Psychiatric Occupational Therapy Approaches for Parents and Children* (Laurette Olson) The Haworth Press, Inc., 2006, pp. 153-156. Single or multiple copies of this article are available for a fee from The Haworth Document Delivery Service [1-800- HAWORTH, 9:00 a.m. - 5:00 p.m. (EST). E-mail address: docdelivery@haworthpress.com].

ing a positive relationship through structured activity in a group setting. Prior research about intervening with parents and their children with mental illness has been based upon expert opinion and anecdotes from clinical practice.

In Chapters 3 through 7, I described a parent-child activity group that I studied through persistent participant observation of the interactions of group participants over an eight-month period and formal and informal interviews of the participants throughout their participation in the group. I described the parents' and children's perspectives about their interactions prior to attending the parent-child activity group and over the course of their participation in the group. The strengths and weaknesses of the leaders' approaches to providing a therapeutic environment and activities for families, and intervening with parents and children as they participated in the group, were examined in depth. What I reported about the participants may resonate with leaders of similar parent-child activity groups. They may find that the descriptions of the participants or the vignettes that I used to illustrate the themes remind them of families with whom they work. They may find that the themes and metathemes are helpful ways to think about my data as well as about their own experiences. What the leaders reported and how I described their interactions with the families may also cause readers to reflect upon how they might optimally lead a parent-child activity group.

I also hope that my descriptions of my activity based group intervention with adolescents with mental illness and their parents and my parent-child intervention with a mother diagnosed with depression may help other clinicians think more deeply about the mental health needs of parents and children related to their co-occupations. There is no research reported in the literature about similar interventions. These are very fruitful areas for research in occupational therapy.

In closing, I would like to highlight what I grew to understand over the course of my clinical work helping parents and children more positively interact in their co-occupations and through my research about a parent-child activity group. Leading a parent-child group requires a high level of leadership skill to be effective in its stated goals. The findings of my study support the findings of prior researchers who have reported that parents and their offspring with mental illness often have interactions that are fraught with conflict, experience limited enjoyment in mutual activity, and have low expectations for family interactions. It is a daunting challenge to help such families discover ways to find enjoyment in each other when they do not expect it.

In the parent-child activity group that I studied, I observed that the leaders learned by doing. The group leaders tended to share pragmatic information among themselves when necessary, but did not reflect together on the process of a particular group or plan the group activities in advance together. Though the group that I observed was helpful to some families, it was not therapeutic for others where the parents and children remained uninvolved with each other. After one leader resigned as a group leader, the remaining leaders shared their feelings of being unsure what to do to help some families. They often did little beyond setting behavioral limits in response to disruptive child behavior and providing materials for the chosen activity for each group.

In Chapter 7, I reflected a great deal on what the alternatives were for intervention and discussed my thoughts about them. I described how viewing parents' and children's participation in the parent-child activity group as cultural voyages may provide a lens for understanding the perspectives of parents and children. It might support the development of collaborative and cooperative relationships between parents and therapists, which is critical for any intervention to be effective.

Parent-child and parent-adolescent activity groups and parent-child occupation-based individual intervention meet different mental health needs and provide a different service than what is typically offered in a psychiatric setting. Parents typically participate in individual and group counseling sessions. Most often, professionals focus on remediating problem behaviors and educating families about mental illness. While these are very important foci, it is also important that families that include a child or parent with mental illness be guided towards learning how to interact in pleasurable and productive ways after hospitalization. So often, these families do not experience the same kind of satisfaction in everyday play and leisure activities that families without a member with mental illness regularly enjoy. Identifying the positive interactions that occur in typical parent-child interaction, but are not occurring in a particular family is as important as identifying the negative behaviors that need to change (Olson, 2001).

Positive and supportive parenting has been linked to the children's adjustment (Pettit, Bates, & Dodge, 1997). Positive and supportive parenting grows in part from feeling confident and effective in parenting one's children and enjoying interactions with those children. Before parents can expect to be effective in limit setting, the first step identified in behavior management plans is for the adult caregiver to successfully engage the child in play. Creating or strengthening a warm relationship between a parent and child positively influences the children's behavior. Children with frequent and high quality positive interaction with a parent will more likely respond to that parent's requests and directions than children who are accustomed to only negative feedback (Foote, Eyberg, & Schuhmann, 1998).

I hope that my work increases readers' awareness of the mental health co-occupational needs and perspectives of children with mental illness and the adults who serve as their primary caregivers, as well as parents with mental illness and the children for whom they serve as primary caregivers. Though interactions between these parents and children are often fraught with conflict, and limited enjoyment of mutual activity is not uncommon, the situation for these families should not be viewed as hopeless. After reading this publication, I hope that readers feel increased empathy for families that include members with mental illness and consider creating occupation-based family groups or individual family interventions.

REFERENCES

Foote, R., Eyberg, S., & Schuhmann, E. (1998). Parent-child interaction approaches to the treatment of child behavior disorders. In T. H. Ollendick & R. J. Prinz (Eds.), *Advances in Clinical Child Psychology* (Vol. 20, pp. 125-151), NY: Plenum Press.
Olson, L. (2001). Child psychiatry in the USA. In L. Lougher (Ed.), *Occupational Therapy for Child and Adolescent Mental Health* (pp. 173-191). Edinburgh: Churchill Livingstone
Pettit, G. S., Bates, J. E. & Dodge, K. A. (1997). Supportive parenting, ecological context, and children's adjustment: A seven-year longitudinal study. *Child Development*, 68, 908-923.

doi:10.1300/J004v22n03_10

Index

For Product Safety Concerns and Information please contact our
EU representative GPSR@taylorandfrancis.com Taylor & Francis
Verlag GmbH, Kaufingerstraße 24, 80331 München, Germany